A Dyslexic Doc's MEMOIRS

Encompassing Breast and Prostate Cancer Detection,
Adultery, Apartheid, Alcoholism, anti-Semitism, E.D.,
Drug Addiction, Dyslexia, Premature Ejaculation,
a Shortbread Recipe, Suicide, Schizophrenia,
a Zulu Murder and More!

Ian Whyte, M.A. (Cantab), M.D.

ZAMA PUBLISHING L.L.C.

ZAMA PUBLISHING L.L.C.
5635 E. Lincoln Drive
Paradise Valley, AZ 85253

The names and identifying details of some individuals
in this book have been changed.

LCCN 2007943759
ISBN-10 0-9802040-0-3
ISBN-13 978-0-9802040-0-1
Copyright information available upon request.

Cover Design: Jim Aiken
Cover Caricature: Mike Fuller
Editor: Jeanne JieAhn
Interior Design: J. L. Saloff
South Africa Map: Susanne Rothwell
Typography: Garamond Premier Pro, Benguiat, and
Loungy and Fontdiner from Fontdinor.com

Note: "Windows 36" refers to Dr. Whyte's photographic memory
of eyes-to-brain and has no relation to the registered software.

First Edition, 2008
Printed on acid free paper.

1.01

This book of memoirs
is dedicated to:

Rosemary, alias "Firefly,"
my wife, my lover, and best friend;

All dyslexics of the world;

Children of the new South Africa,
with hope and good wishes for a brighter future;

To the few of my
misanthropic friends who gave these
memoirs a "thumbs down" prognosis!

And to the many women in
my life who have suffered from
unrequited love, my apologies.

My South Africa

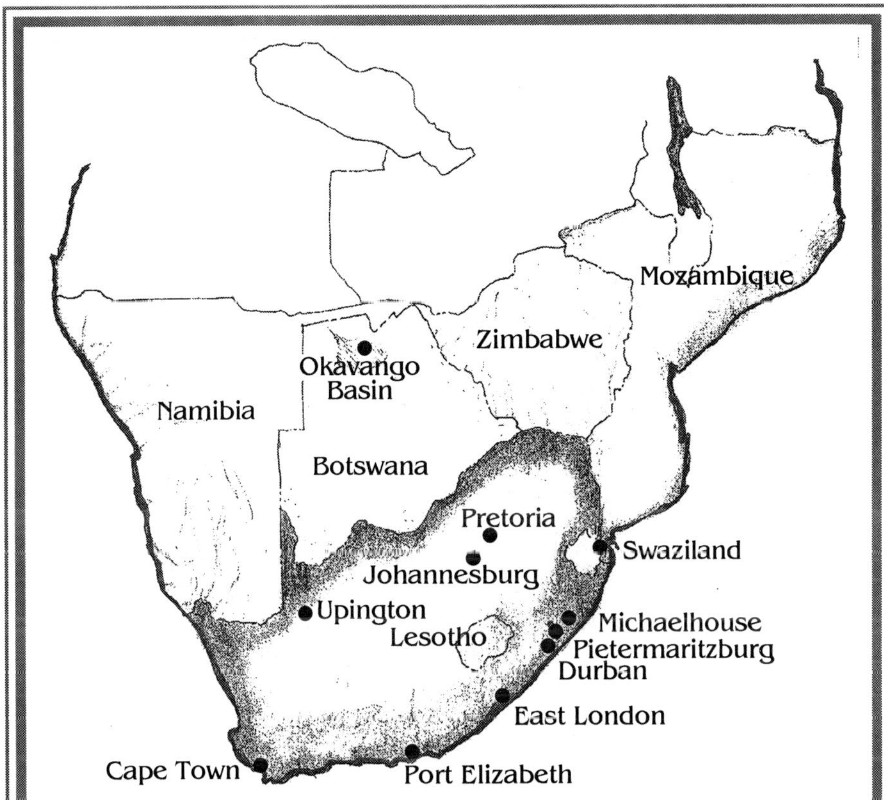

The town of Durban lies on the east coast of South Africa, and has a natural harbor resembling that of San Diego. Various roads lead out of Durban. A six-hour car journey on a superhighway inland will take one to Johannesburg. The highway was built by the South African government to facilitate quick transport of troops to various destinations and allow planes to land in the event insurrection should occur.

The apartheid government was terrified of communism and the possibility that it might be overthrown by the ever-growing elements who violently opposed the racist regime, namely the African National Congress.

Traveling up the north coast of Natal, the road passes through miles of sugar cane plantations. Pythons make their home in the cane fields and keep the rodent population under control. In addition to sugar, "cane spirits" are a popular alcoholic drink. Just ask for "cane," and whatever mix suits your fancy.

At Umhlanga Rocks, the Oyster Box is a most picturesque five-star hotel and restaurant. In season, you can feast on truly delicious oysters, prawns, and lobster tails. If you order prawns, be sure to ask for a spicy "Peri Peri" sauce which had its origins in Portuguese East Africa, precisely the beautiful coastal city of Lourenzo Marquez.

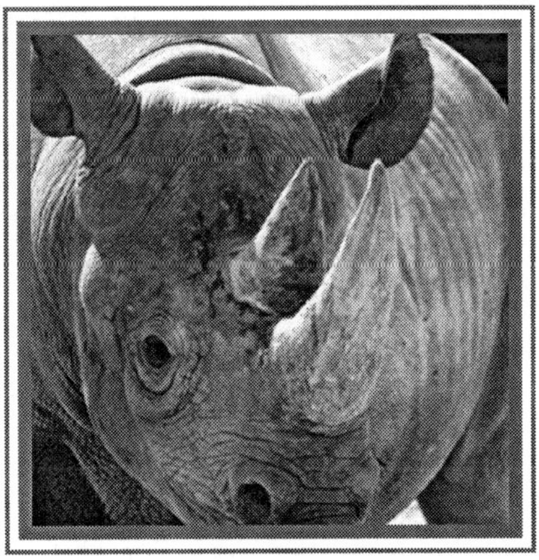

Some distance further north, the road passes through the little town of Gingindlovu (Zulu for "elephant"). A hundred and fifty years ago, elephants roamed these areas as they did in Durban. In fact, some enormous old trees in Durban's Mitchel Park still bear marks of where elephants had rubbed their backs.

Considerably further north is the Hluhluwe Game Reserve, best known of Natal's wildparks. This Zulu name was derived from the monkey ropes growing in the area.

Hluhluwe is the home of the irritable black rhinoceros and the more docile white rhino. I say "docile," but don't kid yourself. These prehistoric beasts have poor eyesight but excellent hearing, and can move faster than you could ever run!

The Hluhluwe Game Reserve is also home to the giraffe, buffalo, zebra, waterbuck, kudu, leopards, cheetah, crocodile and an occasional lion.

Lovely nearby St. Lucia Estuary is eye candy with its huge flocks of colorful flamingos, pelicans, ibis, and herons. If lucky, you may even see a fish-eagle catch a fish! Large numbers of crocodiles and hippopotami make their home at St. Lucia, and can be photographed.

Durban is one of the most beautiful of maritime cities in the world. The subtropical climate can be quite humid in the summer, and vegetation is lush with flowers and trees such as hydrangeas, bougainvillea, frangipani, jacaranda, and flamboyant kaffir boom (coral trees). In the new South Africa, the word "kaffir" (infidel) is not acceptable or tolerated.

Some streets in Durban are lined on both sides with jacarandas. These lovely trees shed their flowers and carpet the streets in blue.

Traveling down the south coast road to Port Edward, one passes a number of seaside resorts—Amanzimtoti, Scottsborough, Uvongo Beach, and Margate. All have beautiful beaches, excellent hotels, and great food.

Just south of Port Edward, Bruce and Lillian Blaise-Smith once owned a quaint bed and breakfast retreat, famous for mixed grill breakfasts. There, private and secluded rondavals (circular, one-story quarters) are a stone's throw from a lovely, secluded beach.

An interesting nearby area of no more than half a square mile resembles a mini-desert. The sand is blood red, as are the rocks. The only such sight I have seen to compare would be the red rocks of Sedona in Arizona (but nowhere as red). I have saved some of these smooth red stones and use them today as paperweights.

The beautiful white sandy beaches of Durban have tempted many tourists from other parts of Africa and other countries. It is a most popular resort town. On North Beach, a miniature train once gave children a fun-filled ride.

Snake Park is an interesting visit. It contains some of the world's most deadly snakes, specifically the green and black mamba. Visit this park only if you are into that sort of thing! If bitten by one of these nasty critters, I do hope you have your last will and testament intact as you will die within minutes unless anti-venom is immediately applied!

There are many five-star hotels on the beachfronts, such as the Edward and Maharani, as well as swimming pools, amusement parks, and probably a MacDonald's or two! When I was a young boy, I enjoyed visiting a favorite ice cream parlor on the beachfront. This parlor sold Eskimo Pies and Twisties (pink spiral, colored cones of ice cream running from top to bottom.) Starting at the top of the Twistie, one must twist off the paper to get at the ice cream—hence its name.

A rickshaw ride along the beachfront is a must, should you be in the area. Rickshaw Boys (adult men) with colorful and elaborate headgear, some with ox horns, will take you for the ride of your life! Periodically and unexpectedly, they will leap from the ground and yell out a blood-curdling Zulu war cry—frightening the hell out of you!

At the end of your rickshaw ride, you can have your photograph taken for a few tickies (three penny pieces). The Rickshaw Boys will say to you in Zulu, "Yabonga Gakoolo" ("Many thanks"). You reply in Zulu, "Hamba Kahle, Sala Kahle" ("Go carefully, stay carefully").

Zulu is a beautiful language. The soulful, melodic music with its repetitive "lullaby-like" refrains is part of the wonderful Zulu nation. Should you ever have the opportunity to listen to the Soweto Choir, for heaven's sake don't miss it! This choir frequently visits the United States and many other countries.

When I was a child living in Durban the population was a little under 600,000, made up almost evenly of whites, blacks (mainly Zulus), and Indians. The Indians originally were brought to South Africa from India to work on the sugar plantations. They were an industrious people, who soon left the plantations for a more lucrative occupation elsewhere.

In 1948, the nationalist government came into power and put apartheid (racism) on the statute books. For the following forty years, they governed South Africa with a ruthless fist of iron. This diabolical, racist regime carried out systematic denigration of the black races in a most inhuman manner.

The white population, on the other hand, comprising about sixty percent Afrikaans and forty percent English, led a spoiled and pampered life. Most white families had at least one servant, and often many more.

For the most part, house servants were treated with kindness by the whites, but not always. Many whites regarded the "kaffirs" as sub-human. Nobody can possibly condone what happened to some of the poor blacks who were interrogated, tortured, and murdered in the apartheid era.

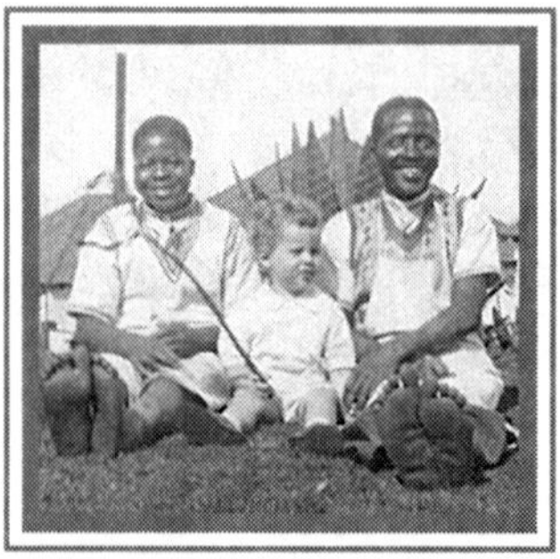
With Nannies, 1932

The Truth and Reconciliation Commission headed by Nobel Prize winner, Rev. Desmond Tutu, went into great detail about the tragic things going on. Wages were appallingly low. Living quarters (kaffir kia's) were cramped and, for the most part, very inadequate.

My family and I did not give the situation a second thought, nor did the vast majority of whites living in South Africa. It was just the way things were meant to be, and that was that!

Natal was mainly English-speaking, but there were many Afrikaners in the northern part of the province. In general, the Afrikaner did not like the English because during the Boer war (1899-1902) many of the Afrikaner women and children died of typhoid and cholera in the British concentration camps.

The white race numbered about five million, and the black race (consisting of many different tribes) around thirty million. Zulus lived mainly in Natal and numbered around seven million. The Zulus are a beautiful people, proud, good-looking with white shiny teeth, and magnificent singing voices.

My mother often sang Zulu lullabies, guaranteed to put me to sleep. "Thina sobabili, sotanda indunduma" was sung over and over again (translated, "Your daddy and mommy, both the two of us, love you heaps.")

This country I have described is where I was born, a little dyslexic white boy, spoiled rotten.

My parents came from humble beginnings. Dad was born in a little village called Upington, in the northwest of the Cape Province, bordering on the Kalahari Desert. There, the climate was desert, with dry hot days and cold nights. It was a wonderful citrus area, almost identical to the Southwest United States. Not far away were the diamond fields of Southwest Africa and the Augrabies Water Falls.

Dad's parents were dirt-poor, and Jewish. His first language was Afrikaans, and the Afrikaner is generally quite anti-Semitic. The Goldbergs did not have an easy time of it running their small hotel and bottle store (liquor store).

Possibly the only Jew accepted by the Afrikaners, was Okkie Geffin, a Springbok rugby player with a phenomenal kick!

Rugby in South Africa is a religion, so I imagine the Afrikaners felt Okkie must have passed the muster and was just okay, in spite of being Jewish.

My mother was born in Scotland in 1900, and at the age of seven she and her family moved to South Africa. Her father was a baker, and an alcoholic, as were his 14 brothers. They were all born in Scotland of teetotaling parents. I imagine the Scottish climate might have had something to do with that!

Granny and Mom had a miserable time living with my grandfather, James Weymes Whyte. They often had to fish him out of pubs and haul him home, dead drunk. On one such occasion, they found a dead bird in his pocket. He had wanted to take it home for my mother—presumably, when it was still alive!

The story goes that my granny, who for years had to put up with grandpa's God-awful drinking, locked him in a room with a bottle of Scotch. She left him there for a considerable time, warning him that if even one drop was missing from the bottle, he was history. (This was many years before Alcoholics Anonymous.)

Well, as the story goes, granny returned later to find that not one drop of liquor had been taken! (How could she count drops in the liquor bottle?) Anyway, Grandpa never drank again! He went on to become the mayor of Newcastle Natal, and had a thriving bakery business as well. One hears of such success stories, but they are scarce.

Granny was an excellent cook. Her two specialties were fudge and pancakes. Over the years, we often attempted to follow her fudge recipe—but it was never quite the same!

Grandpa loved birds, and pigeons often flew up to their windowsill where grandpa always fed them. One pigeon had a broken foot and was affectionately named by grandpa as Crippled Dick.

The last time I saw him, grandpa and granny were living at the Waverley Hotel in Durban. He was eighty years old, and a diabetic. I recall the holes he had cut in his shoes to accommodate large bunions. I also recall grandpa's pipe rack sitting atop the mantel with many different shaped pipes. They smelled awful! Strange how one remembers such small incidents of long ago.

Mother had a twin brother, Robert. He was a man with a fine baritone singing voice, but also had an addiction to alcohol and cigarettes. Robert died at age forty-two of lung cancer. It was sad to see him dying, skin and bones, a shadow of his former self. (In those days, the connection between smoking and lung cancer was not recognized.)

Robert had two sons, William and Garret. William was a year or two older than me. He started at the University of Cape Town Medical School, but soon quit because students were required to dissect a dogfish, frog, or rabbit. This turned William off. He could not go through with it, and William was put off medicine forever!

My cousin William ultimately entered the ministry, joining a silent order in England. He stayed in the ministry for seventeen years, but then came out and married a woman from Southern Rhodesia (now called Zimbabwe). She was some twenty years his junior. They had one little girl named Dawn.

William recounted some of his experiences in Southern Rhodesia while in the ministry. He said he was often required to go to outlying farms to give communion to the farmers. Those drives were dangerous and meant white knuckles from gripping the steering wheel, because the roads were full of land mines! But the Lord must have been with William—he was never blown up.

These were the times when Ian Smith's government fought the terrorists (Ters), Mugabie and Company. Robert Gabriel Mugabe was born in 1924. He ruled the country with an iron fist until 1980 when he became Prime Minister, and later First Executive President. The government was corrupt, ruthlessly crushing political opposition and often taking away land from productive white farmers.

Such mismanagement (and more) resulted in the economic collapse of the country and massive starvation over the last ten years. Zimbabwe has the highest inflation rate in the world (2220 percent!), and is a classic example of what can befall a once beautiful and prosperous country.

Ian Smith prophesized that Rhodesia would be "buggered" if the blacks took over, and that is just what seems to be happening. Eight out of every ten Zimbabweans are jobless today.

It is extremely disturbing to hear that when the Commonwealth moved to expel Mugabe, South Africa actually helped to block them! South Africa also thwarted attempts to place Mugabe's atrocities on the agenda of the UN Security Council and the UN Human Rights Committee.

My cousin, Dawn, attended the University of Cape Town, and she and I once began an e-mail relationship. Her mother intercepted one of her "Uncle Ian's e-mails" which she viewed as unacceptably cheeky. That was the end of our e-mail relationship. (I suppose when one is married to a man like William—who had been in a silent religious order for seventeen years—one looks at things differently.)

Garrett, mother's twin brother's son, was a ne'er-do-well and ran into all kinds of trouble with the law. The last time I saw Garrett, he was in jail for stealing a Durban VIP's motorcar.

I had not seen Garrett in years but I was most curious to see what the inside of a jail looked like, so I decided to pay a visit. My black sheep cousin stood behind the bars with a sickly psychopathic smile on his face as I approached him. We did not have much to talk about, and he died some years later under somewhat mysterious circumstances. William would never give me any details.

Mother had three other brothers, all of whom were alcoholics. The youngest, Ross, once ran Whyte's Bakery into the ground. Jack was the oldest and had an illegitimate child—a female—whom I have never met. Most likely, I have a cousin roaming around the new South Africa—somewhere!

My mother became a nurse at Grey's Hospital in Pietermaritzburg, and it was there she met dad. (Dad had managed to get into the University of Cape Town Medical School. He had to finance his way through medical school by working nights as a demonstrator in the anatomy school.)

Dad's handwriting was so bad that his examiners could not read what he had written, and had to bring him back again and again to read his answers to them. In retrospect, this may have been a manifestation of dyslexia. From then on, dad learned to print.

Many years later, when I lived in the United States, I received a letter from dad. His letter came from South Africa shortly before he died, and it arrived in the U.S. a few days after his death. His printing was beautiful, and I have kept this letter ever since as a memento.

Dad's younger brother, Roger Goldberg, was left-handed and a tremendous tennis player. He became a very successful lawyer in Port Elizabeth, and also the mayor. He also bred racehorses, and was without a doubt my favorite uncle.

My Uncle Roger always had a supply of biltong for me (sun-dried salted meat), usually Springbok. He would often say, "Sherry, wine, and baby clothes—that's where all my money goes." Strange how one remembers these things!

Roger's daughter, Dorothy, is married to the botany professor at University Cape Town. She and I correspond periodically, but no risqué e-mails this time!

In 1933, a near-miracle occurred. My parents changed their name from Goldberg to Whyte (spelled with a "Y", please!). Whyte was my mother's maiden name and I still have the official change-of-name document with its green tassel. The posh new name was my passport into Michaelhouse, a very prestigious school in South Africa, and later to Pembroke College, Cambridge. It was also my father's entry card to a variety of international places which, with the name Goldberg, he would have had difficulty obtaining.

The reason behind the name change, as the story goes, was the existence of another "Harry Goldberg, MD," residing in Durban—one who was up to shady practices. (None of dad's brothers or sisters ever bothered to change their names.)

So there you have an introduction to my lineage. As you can see, our family was not exactly unblemished or aristocratic. In fact, many of us could be called dysfunctional renegades. I am not sure I would have it any other way!

The moving finger writes, and
having writ, moves on.
Nor all thy piety nor wit
shall lure it back to cancel half a line,
nor all thy tears wash out a word of it.

The Rubaiyat,
Omar Khayyam

South Africa

- 1930 -

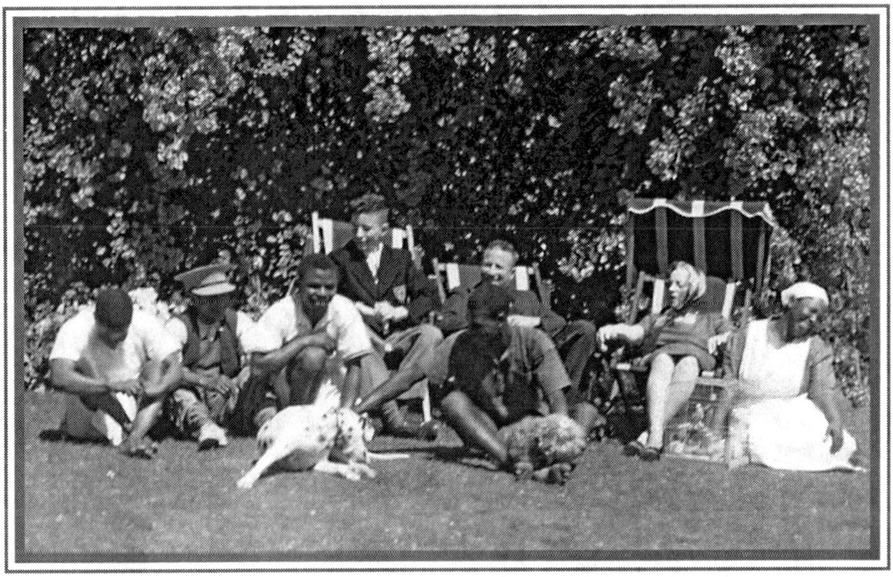

We had so much; they had so little.

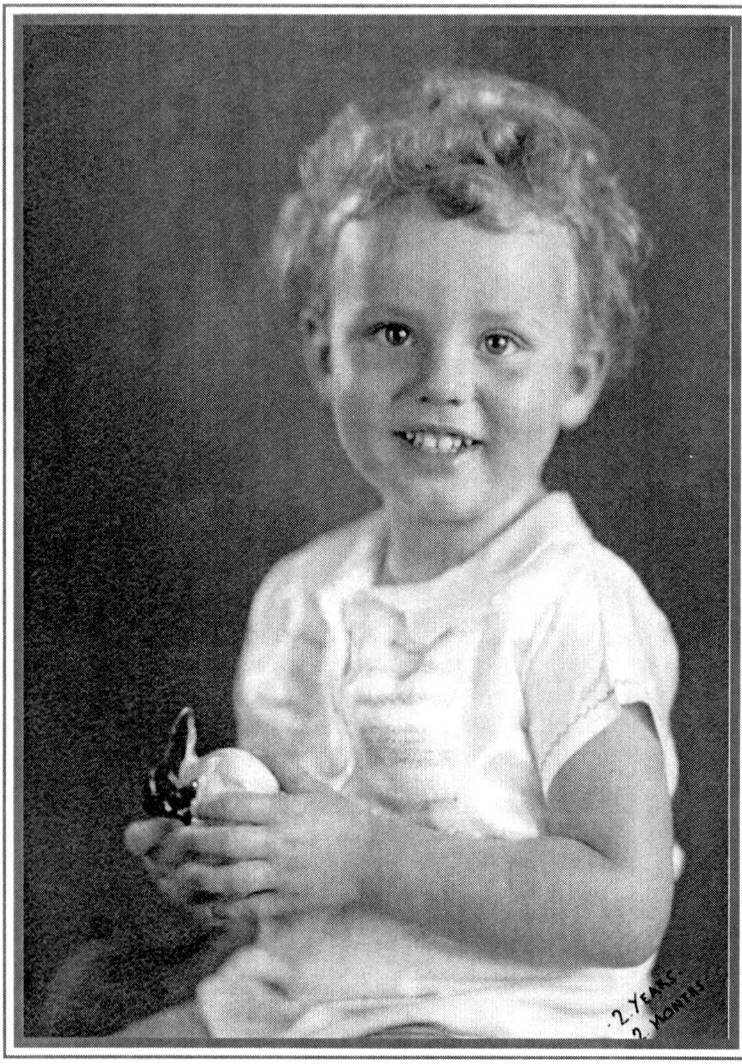

The Author!

A piece of chalk went sailing across the classroom and hit me dead center on my forehead.

It was "day one" in Mr. Lewin's reading class when I first entered junior school in 1936. I was the unlucky recipient of Mr. Lewin's sullen frown.

"Read! " he shouted.

I stared at the simple sentence in the textbook ("I see a kitty, a kitty sees me").

"Kitty a see I," I said, hopefully.

"No, no, no! " shouted Mr. Lewin, as he reached for his chalk.

Squirming uncomfortably, I tried again. "Me sees kitty a?"

The chalk went flying, but this time I dodged it!

Things went from bad to worse, and thus began my lifelong bloody struggle with reading, writing, and spelling!

I do not believe the word "dyslexia" existed in those days. If it did, not too many people knew what it meant. Even today, many teachers are unable to recognize a student with dyslexia.

Born left-handed, my parents believed I had a "left-handed disability." In fact, I was afflicted with this God-awful disability from birth. It was decided by mom and dad to change me into a "right-handed" little boy—which only created merry hell with my reading and writing. Not only could I not read, but I began to "mirror write" which involved reversal of letters and numbers.

Dyslexics do not outgrow their condition—reading and writing tend to remain tough obstacles for life. Dyslexia can be mild to moderate, or severe, and mine was exceedingly severe. To this very day, I am plagued by my dyslexic condition.

There are certified dyslexia testing specialists available. If you suspect your child might be dyslexic, it is imperative to have testing done by such an ethical individual as soon as possible. When I was growing up, there were no such services. Not being able to read closes the door on a world of information. The dyslexic is often labeled as dumb, careless or lazy—a most unfortunate stigma!

As a young schoolboy, my parents, Mr. Lewin, and I did not have the slightest idea of the cause and magnitude of my problem. Of course, Mr. Lewin could have cared less!

(The causes of dyslexia appear to involve genetic chromosomal abnormalities, together with some faulty brain wiring. One is born with it—to a lesser or greater extent.)

On a chilly winter's morning at 4:30 a.m. on August 22, 1930 in Durban, South Africa, I made my noisy entrance into the world, bum (buns) first. A most appropriate arrival for a dyslexic! In the years to follow, I would often get things back to front!

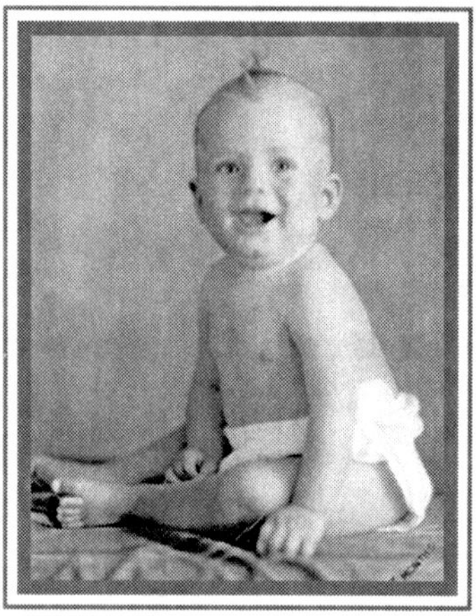

The Author

My birth certificate states my name to be Ian Goldberg-Whyte. I was a nice little half-Jewish baby, as my father was Jewish and my mother Scottish. Our home in Durban had all the comforts, complete with servants. I was a pampered only-child until my brother Peter was born nine years later.

Durban, South Africa, is one of the most picturesque and beautiful maritime cities in the world on the east coast of Southern Africa—a bewitching, sun-drenched port on the Indian Ocean. Durban's subtropical climate can be quite humid in the summer months. The vegetation is lush with flowers and trees such as hydrangeas, bougainvillea, frangipani, and jacaranda. Durban is very much like San Diego, California. This is where I grew up—one spoiled little brat!

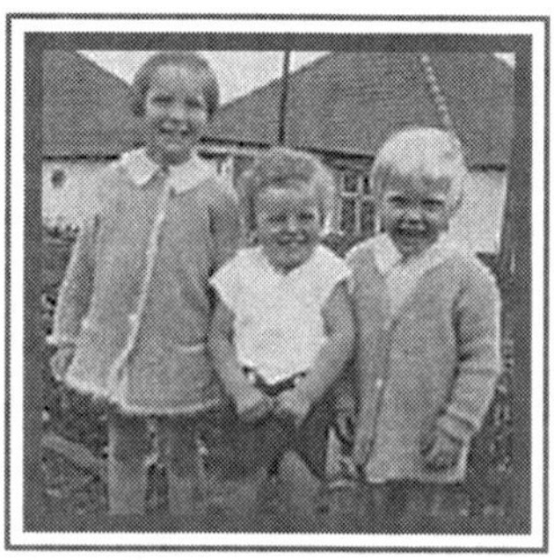

The Ladies Man

Looking at faded old photographs today, those taken before age six with a Baby Brownie camera (remember those?) in 1933, 1934 and 1935 do not bring back memories. The pics simply portray a little boy with parents, the ever-present black nanny, or neighborhood boys and girls—but I have no memories. I was about seven years old when my photographic memory came into sharp focus. This blessing allowed me to adjust to my dyslexia, and was an absolute God-send.

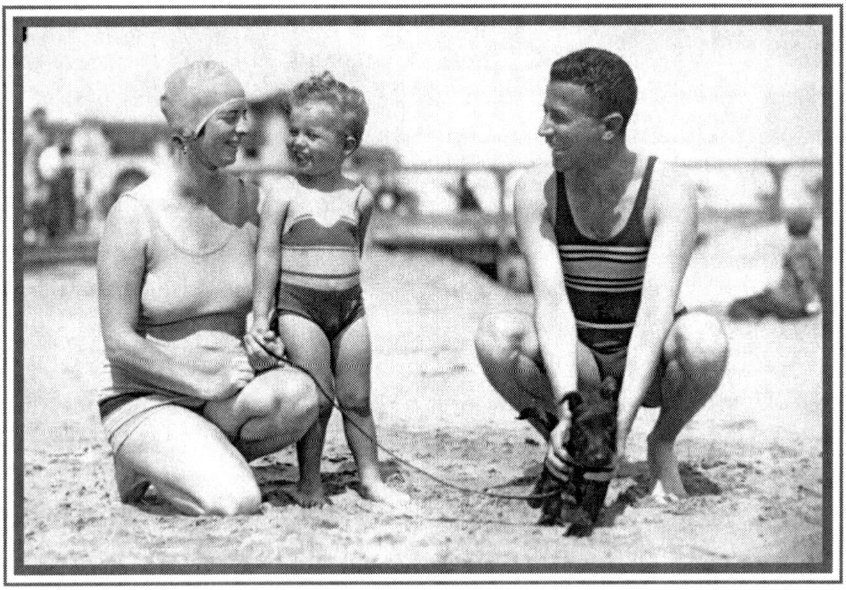

Mom and Dad, Durban Beach, 1932

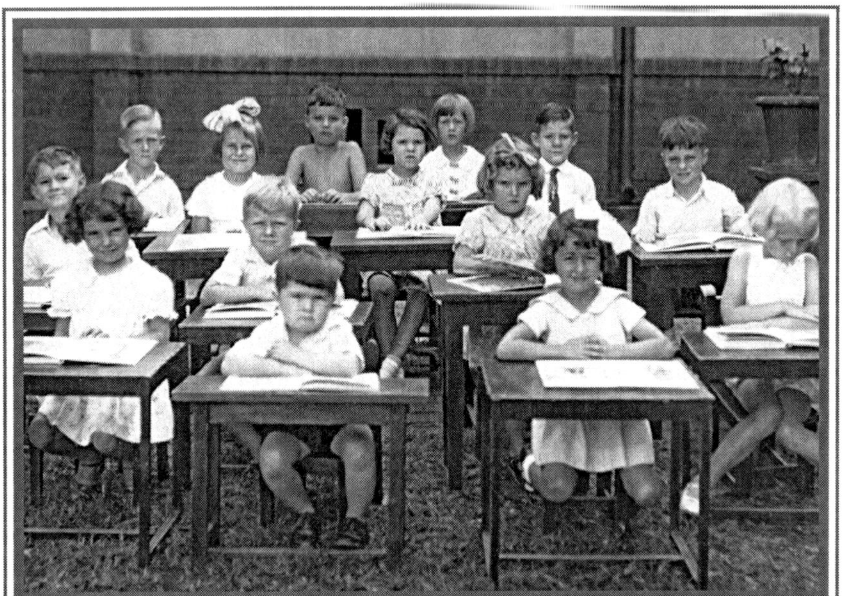

Sitting in back row with no top

My parents strongly believed in the philosophy of Mr. A.S. Neil, head of the Summer Hill School in England. This highly progressive school believed that children should be allowed to do as they please! In my parents' infinite wisdom, I was allowed to do exactly that. Just what I pleased!

Sitting at the top of our staircase at home, I had great fun throwing "45" gramophone records down the stairs—record after record, with no parental retribution. One snapshot shows me at my nursery school, sitting topless, while the other children had to wear tops.

I once bit a teacher on her forearm because she had asked me to get out of the sandbox when I did not want to. I then threw sand into her new permanent wave hairdo. Unlike my parents, the teacher soundly walloped me! Such a dear little boy was I!

Lizzie is in one of my snaps. She was a white mother's helper who must have been in her late teens. Lizzie lived with us in our home, and when I was about age twelve she introduced me to the ways of the flesh!

There is a snap of my very dear friend, Peter, whom I met in 1933. He lived next door and was three or four years older than me. Peter was of Scandinavian descent—a good looking, blond, blue-eyed young lad. We have retained our friendship to this day, and still acknowledge each other's birthdays.

Peter read stories to me provided I would tickle the soles of his feet. Since I could not read, this was a sweet deal. We often rode in his boxcart to the Varsity Tea Room, a quarter mile down Manning Road. There we bought chewing gum (Wrigley or P.K., spearmint or peppermint) for a penny a packet, containing three pieces.

Many years later, I visited the wealthy Wrigley Mansion in the Arizona Biltmore Estates and Mr. Wrigley's incredible home on Catalina Island. I was impressed, and couldn't help but think that Mr. Wrigley must have sold many packets of chewing gum!

When I was a very young lad, my friends and I decided to form a so-called "enema club," and we named it "Elephant 8." It is possible that elephants did in fact once live there, eating the trees, but I don't think it had anything to do with the name of our club. Heaven alone knows how we came up with the "8" since there were only six of us—five boys and one girl, Susie.

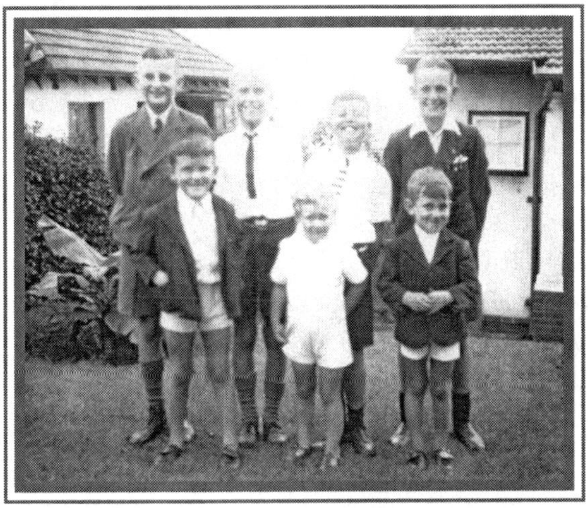

Members of the Elite Elephant 8, Enema Club

Basil was somewhat older than the rest of us. He suggested that we only allow Susie to join our club if she showed us her private parts. So we all gathered around as she very obligingly removed her panties. Susie immediately became a lifetime member of Elephant 8.

There were some deadly snakes in the bush where our club meetings took place, and it is amazing that we were never bitten. The underbrush had been cleared, and only the monkey vines remained—rope-like structures between the trees. We sat on these for the enemas. Granted, they could be a bit tippy! Our only audience, a few African gray monkeys, must have been more than a little curious at what they were seeing.

It was I who produced the enema apparatus, which consisted of a six-foot long tube and a water container. These items were not difficult to get hold of since, in that era, the enema was a cure for a multitude of conditions. (Coffee enemas were not yet known in the sub-Saharan countries.)

The exercise was to fill the can with water, insert the end of the tube into one's anus while sitting on a monkey rope, and then hold the water in as long as possible. Then, with great force, expel it to see how far we could shoot the stream. Basil won almost every time. He was about twelve years old, the leader, and bigger than the rest of us.

Susie did not last long in "Elephant 8." Basil wanted to put the enema tube somewhere else, and she screamed at him in Afrikaans, "Ag, Sis man, Voetsek" ("Bugger off, you dirty bastard! "). With that, she pulled up her panties and left the club forever.

(I saw Susie many years later at the University of Cape Town. We did not bring up the subject of Elephant 8.)

The reputation of our club had spread, and other boys were most anxious to join. We soon had possibly nine or ten members. One new arrival was Larry Warmback—of course, we immediately called him Larry Coldfront. I recall how Larry's father played the xylophone so beautifully. On many a summer's evening, his soothing melodies wafted to our homes in deeply fragrant air when the frangipanis were in bloom.

Another new arrival was Colin Visser, whose privates amazingly resembled a skinny rainworm. His nickname became "Shongololo" (Zulu for "rainworm"). Colin would one day enroll in RADA (Royal Academy of Dramatic Arts in London, England), and become a member of the gay community. He was also to be my best man at my marriage in August, 1954.

Well, the club came to a grinding halt when mother walked in on an Elephant 8 club meeting. I think she had been suspicious of the various goings-on, and had spotted the entrance to our hideout.

The meeting was in full swing and the winner was about to be declared, when in walked mother. Talk about a shocker! She confiscated the enema tube and container, and straightaway sent us home. But mother was also a free spirit and she assured us that she would not inform the other parents—unless we tried to revive the club.

For six years, my father had been a doctor in general practice in Durban—surgery, obstetrics, gynecology, and everything else. It had become too much for him. He was having recurring chest pains and would inhale amyl nitrate (which stank bloody awful, much like dirty feet!) from a crushed vial for relief. Amyl nitrate was used many years later by hippies to enhance orgasm.

So in 1936 dad went to England to study for a DA (Diploma in Anesthesiology). There was no specialist training for anesthesiology at that time in South Africa.

Dad boarded a luxurious Pan Am flying boat in Durban. The flight took a week to get to London and it would come down on the Great Lakes of Central Africa at night to refuel, and to let the passengers have a good night's sleep. During the day the aircraft flew low enough to allow passengers to view the amazing wildlife below—an incredible journey.

A few months after my father departed for England my mother, Lizzie (mother's helper), and I went to visit him. We set sail on the "Bloemfontein Castle" from Cape Town, a voyage lasting three weeks.

Mother was blond and pretty, and frequently wore colored polka-dot dresses with a square low-cut neckline. (When she pruned hydrangeas in our garden at home and leaned forward, it was obvious she wore no bra!) We were not onboard long before mother had the attention of a naval officer onboard the ship.

Sam was from Holland, tall and good-looking, and he spoke with a funny accent. He seemed to like mother and made her a small replica of a Spanish galleon in exquisite detail. After she died in 1966, I received this galleon and kept it in my office for many years.

One afternoon I walked into our cabin to find mother and Sam kissing in bed! I remember Sam had a lot of black curly hair on his back, and he seemed quite aback taken at seeing me! Mother showed no embarrassment and simply said, "Its okay, darling, just go upstairs and I'll get you an ice cream in a jiffy."

In London, it was good to see dad again. Actually I hardly knew my father since he worked so hard. His schedule had always been to arise early, and then do what all old-fashioned general practitioners did—everything. It would be late in the evenings before he returned home.

During this visit to England, my mother took Lizzie and me on a side trip to Germany. We visited Berlin—I recall the fast moving trains, and eating German toffee. We rode a train to the Zugspitzer, world famous German ski resort near Garmisch. It is Germany's highest mountain and host to the 4th Winter Olympics in 1936—the first Olympics to have downhill skiing.

While at the Zugspitzer, we watched several dozen German soldiers practice their skiing. They were dressed in white ski uniforms and were excellent skiers. We had no idea that in just a few years these young men would be fighting in the Second World War, killing our countrymen.

Shortly before departing England, mother and I visited the famously

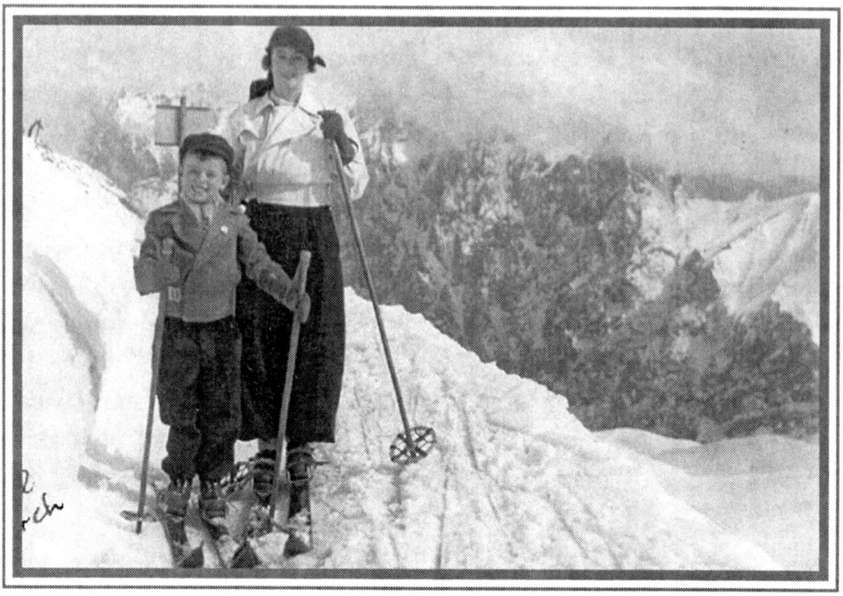

Mother and me, 1936

progressive residential school, Summer Hill, founded by A.S. Neill in 1927. This school encouraged children to recite Shakespeare to cows, enjoy communal nude sunbathing, and anything else that may occur to them. Mother appeared to be very impressed with the permissive and yet progressive nature of the school, but she already had many of her own liberated ideas, long before visiting Summer Hill.

Surprisingly, the founder's daughter Zoe Neill Readhead, who now runs the school, introduced—of all things—Rules! She had reportedly told the London Times that children were coming from homes where they were being overly indulged.

Following a brief visit to Trafalgar Square to feed the pigeons, mother and I said goodbye to my hard-studying dad and returned to South Africa.

In retrospect, one wonders if one's parents were good or bad. Mine were different, very different, but I knew they both loved me. They were very much ahead of their time and would have possibly fit in better thirty years later.

We returned to South Africa once again on the Bloemfontein Castle, with the same crew. Sam was pleased to see us or, more precisely pleased to see mom. This time I was to share Lizzie's cabin since my mother needed her beauty sleep.

There were many children on the ship, and I had plenty of playmates. The captain once organized a fancy dress costume children's party for us, and I dressed up as Mickey Mouse.

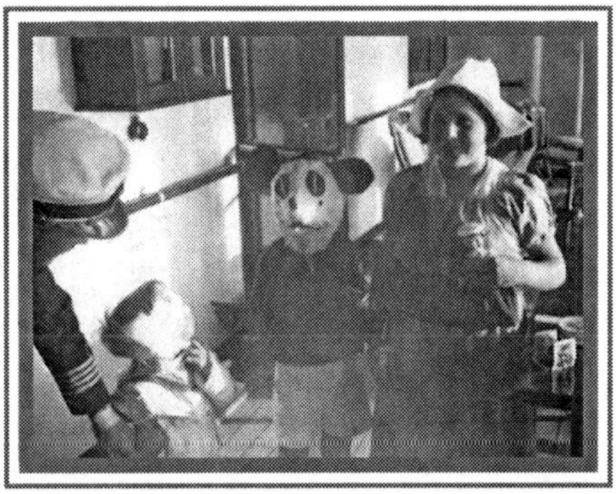

Mickey Mouse Fancy Dress Party and Sam (Mother's good friend)

Toward the end of the party, I decided to hide behind a big chair where I remained hidden for quite a long time. Nobody could find me. They thought I might have fallen overboard, and people became frantic. All hell broke loose in the search.

Finally, curious about all the commotion, I poked my Mickey Mouse head out of hiding long enough to take a look, but then I was discovered. This was one of the very few times in my childhood when mother lost her temper and walloped me hard. So much for Summer Hill School's laissez-faire!

Dad eventually returned from England with his hard-earned diploma, and became the first specialist anesthesiologist in South Africa. He later received the highest possible degree in anesthesiology, both in the U.K. and in the United States.

At Natal Medical School, a black medical school for Africans, Indians, and colored students, dad was Professor of Anesthesiology. In time, he also became President of the South African Medical Association.

My dad had come a long way! It would be a hard act to follow for me—his dyslexic son who could not read or write.

There are four things I remember about Mr. Lewin, my junior school reading teacher: 1) He made my life miserable; 2) he could whistle with his mouth closed; 3) he could throw chalk with remarkable accuracy; and 4) he was a complete son of a bitch.

Clifton Preparatory School was located on Lambert Road in Durban. When I entered junior school, profoundly dyslexic, in 1936, Mr. Lewin would pick on me without mercy, calling me stupid. I was the recipient of his multiple barrages of chalk. He blamed me for disrupting his class. It became so bad that I felt nauseated in the mornings, and did not want to attend school.

Mother spoke to Mr. Lewin, but this only made things worse. My "left-handed disability," as my mother put it, did not interest him.

Finally, mother arranged special reading lessons for me with a very kind and gentle woman, Mrs. Hanna Ball. Mrs. Ball took a piece of cardboard and cut out a narrow strip to accommodate three or four words only. The rest of the words on the page were blocked out. Unfortunately, this did not help as it did not stop my reading from right to left.

Many years later (1971), I attended a speed-reading class in Montreal given by Ms. Evelyn Wood, and this class resulted in wonderful improvements. My reading went from 100 wpm with next to no recall, to 500 wpm with excellent recall.

The secret was in using the index finger as a pacer, moving it from left to right just below the written line. By letting one's eyes follow the tip of the index finger, word repetition was prevented (going back). This simple technique is also helpful for slow readers or those with other reading difficulties.

Mr. Lewin badgered me into the third grade. But it was in third grade that I discovered, quite by pure chance, that nature had provided me with an advantage to compensate for my dyslexia—literally, a photographic memory! I found that I could look at certain words or pictures in minute detail, and then transfer this information to my brain for future reference. Ian's "Windows 36" Copy and Paste! What a find!

This photographic memory must have been there all along, but it seemed to pop out of nowhere! Once discovered, I was able to skip a grade and went from fourth to sixth grade in one year. Mr. Lewin was finally out of my life forever!

One of Mr. Lewin's favorite punishments was to make me copy 500 lines in a copybook. I cannot remember how many times I had to carry out this exercise, but it certainly stopped my mirror writing and made my writing almost legible most of the time!

After Mr. Lewin and I parted company, junior school years went by quickly.

John Sinclair, a student in my class, had also skipped a grade. I was never able to achieve more than John, much as I tried. John always came first, and I second! In later years, he became internationally famous as a judge. He was brilliant. When he eventually died, John's obituary honored him with an outstanding write-up.

In my junior school years the accidental discovery that my brain, dyslexic though it may be, could act as a computer, was something I did not understand. But something was definitely working for me! My mirror writing and the reversal of letters and numbers was a situation that was corrected by the old-fashioned copybook.

For those who do not know what a copybook is, it is a book that assists one to improve their writing. By copying over the light print, many times, many lines, many pages, I was able to correct my mirror writing and reversal of numbers. This was the only good thing to come out of my relationship with that little squirt Mr. Lewin! This was his punishment for what he believed was my disruptive behavior in his reading class.

Later in my high school years, at Michaelhouse, I would review the past ten years of matriculation examination questions and memorize the answers. This was done by laboriously copying the answers from textbooks, one word at a time. Having to contend with my eyes repeatedly wanting to go back [from right to left] rereading the word I had just read. I would copy down the answers in my own appalling handwriting, the prelude to pasting the answers in my memory bank.

This involved considerable time and "stick-to-it-ive-ness." By writing down these answers over and over again I was able to get them just right. I wrote the answers in a black book, approximately six by nine inches. This book I carried into my examinations in my brain's computer. This book contained all the answers to the last ten years of examination questions. These questions would sooner or later recur, as they were very important questions.

Looking back many years later, I realized what was happening. My eyes (Ian`s Windows 36) were the conduit to my brain`s computer. This involved complex hand (writing down) eye (photographing) coordination in order for me to be able to paste this information securely into my memory so later I could reproduce the data on demand. It was virtually like taking your textbooks into the examinations!

At Cambridge I got a black board and used different color chalks. The backboard was essentially a monitor, and I was able to photograph the images. This was my visual aid to success.

My photographic memory enabled me to succeed in high school, Pembroke College Cambridge, and later in my clinical years at St. Thomas' Hospital in London. Please do not think for a minute that I could photograph Grey's Anatomy into my memory bank, all 1542 pages! No way! However, I could summarize important pages on my blackboard, using colored chalk, and then commit these images to my memory.

Today the curser on my Dell computer monitor guides my eye from left to right. Essentially, in my earliest school days I was using a blackboard much as a monitor with my eyes and uniquely wired brain as a homegrown computer.

Dyslexics often have excellent long-term memories for experiences, locations, and faces. We think primarily with images and feelings. These compensatory skills can often be used to great advantage. To go into an examination with the answers to all the questions imaged in my brain was quite uncanny. Even spooky! I was able to complete examinations long before many of my contemporaries! (I confess this proved true for me in all but one examination—but it was a big one!)

My writing, on the other hand, was a different story. On occasion, I still have difficulty reading my own writing, and I am disinclined to read, even to this day. Subtitles in movies are totally out, since they disappear too quickly and I am not able to use my finger as a pacer.

Exciting, fast-paced novels interest me as reading material. One such novel (641 pages!) prompted me to write my own book of memoirs. "White Thorn" was authored by Bryce Courtenay, a magnificent storyteller! Bryce was born in South Africa and now lives in Australia. He is the author of many wonderful books.

Mr. Tim Sutcliffe arrived at Clifton as the new principal, along with his very pretty wife, Yolande (who I secretly lusted for!). Mr. Sutcliffe introduced the class to the works of George Bernard Shaw and many other fascinating authors. He read to us and imitated the accents of the various characters, which sparked interest in our young minds. Encouraged, my parents bought me the complete leather bound works of George Bernard Shaw, with high hopes of whetting my interest. But I never read them.

A strict disciplinarian, Mr. Sutcliffe had no mercy when Andrew Black and I were disruptive in one of his classes. Pulling us out of class, he took us to his office. There he gave us four strokes on our bare bottoms with an old English cane. It hurt like hell! The marks on our bottoms remained for many weeks.

My mother was furious at Mr. Sutcliffe for this incident, but it did me little actual harm. It certainly was radical change from my usual permissive upbringing, and likely did me some good!

Another teacher comes to mind—one Pat Dakin, who taught Art. Ms. Dakin was a captivating redhead. She was sexy, and was far ahead of her time with her low-cut blouses and mini-skirts. Many a pencil was dropped in front of her desk by young boys with healthy hormones!

Talking about this kind of thing reminds me of seeing the Barnum and Bailey Circus. It was my fervent hope that the elastic in the young female trapeze artists' panties would break! It never happened.

When father decided to change our name from Goldberg to Whyte (because of the other Dr. Harry Goldberg in Durban, who was up to shady practices), Durban was still a small town. And so, merely changing one's name did not make one "un-Jewish." The fact that I was only half Jewish and could, in theory, wear a kilt (since my mother was Scottish) mattered not at all!

One little bastard in school by the name of Drain (odd name, isn't it?) commented one day, "Ian is a damned Jew."

I told my parents, but what could they do? This was my first taste of anti-Semitism, but not my last.

Since only a few people were aware of my name change, I was often privy to anti-Semitic remarks and jokes. This made me realize that anti-Semitism is alive and well, even among many well-educated people.

By age 12, my hormones had kicked in big time. I began to notice that our white nanny, Lizzie, was not exactly ugly. The keyhole opposite one end of our bathroom gave me a private view of Lizzie taking a bath. Her pink nipples protruding through the soapy water were an absolutely hypnotizing sight.

My parents were out the first time Lizzie came into my room. I had been having fantasies of being caught by a tribe of beautiful Amazon women, striped naked, tied up and slowly masturbated! Why a beautiful Amazon woman would want to have anything to do with a twelve year-old boy boggles the mind. But such was the fantasy when Lizzie entered my room. I was terribly embarrassed, and ashamed at being caught, but Lizzie said nothing. She simply leaned over and gently kissed it. Within seconds, I had climaxed.

Later, I would discover that this was the birth of "primary premature ejaculation," a most troublesome and distressing condition that plagued me for years, through university days and on into two marriages. This is such an important subject and so rarely discussed. As an addendum at the end of the book, I will put on my doctor's white coat and tell you everything you ever wanted to know about primary and secondary PE, but were too embarrassed to ask.

Ineffectual sex with Lizzie continued for the following year until I went to boarding school at Michaelhouse. It still remains a mystery to me why Lizzie ever bothered with me since she had a grown-up boyfriend, Rupert, but I was not about to complain. Today such behavior with a minor would subject Lizzie to arrest and prosecution.

Rupert was much older than Lizzie. He had red hair and pale blue eyes, and always impressed me as being a bit of a wimp. He worked at a refrigeration plant down by the Durban docks, and one day asked my friend, Peter, and me if we would like to see the place.

It was a Saturday, and we arrived there about 12:30 p.m. The three of us stepped into one of the huge refrigerated storage rooms—freezing cold and used primarily to store frozen fish—when Rupert accidentally slammed the big heavy door shut! With no interior handle on the door, we could not get out!

We banged on the freezer door and screamed bloody murder, but all of the employees in the plant had gone home for the weekend. There was no one around to hear our frantic cries for help. It was a damned terrifying experience!

As luck would have it, and after what seemed an eternity, a woman employee returned to the plant to retrieve a forgotten something in her office. She heard our frantic knocking, and came to our rescue.

This incident was only one of many narrow escapes in my life. An orthopedic surgeon friend of mine, Big Jim, once appropriately referred to me as "the cat," with nine lives.

My mother had several miscarriages before my brother was born in 1939. I recall her bleeding profusely in the bathroom, and it frightened me.

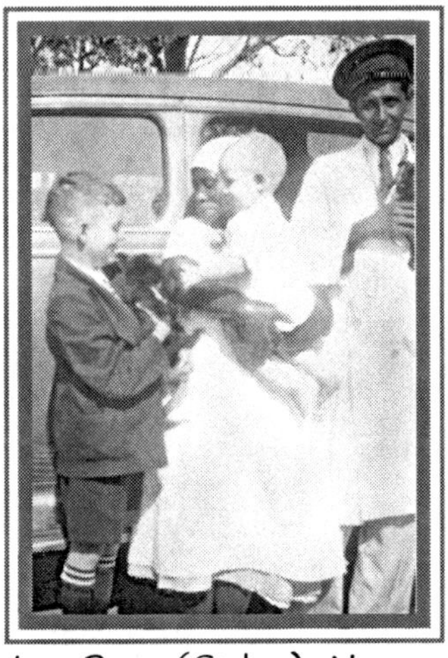

Ian, Peter (Sinker), Nanny, and Gannas

Peter was born on August 13, 1939. We nicknamed him "Sinker" because during my mother's pregnancy she was teased that if she were to go swimming, she would sink. Peter had a little blue rabbit stuffed toy that he carried wherever he went. Much like a security blanket, I would presume.

With a difference of nine years in our age, I essentially grew up as a single child. Still, I was proud of Sinker, and happy that I acquired a brother.

Peter grew up and attended the

University of Natal where he studied Law. He received a first class pass in Zulu, which enabled him to defend Zulu clients during the Apartheid era—something few lawyers were prepared or willing to do. He then went on to Cambridge University to further study Law, and again received a first-class pass.

After Peter married, his Czechoslovakian wife, Sarah, was uncomfortable living in South Africa. Both of them felt conditions there were deteriorating, so they moved to England—much to my mother's disappointment. By then, Mother had both sons out of the country.

In England, Peter joined the British Government's Public Prosecution Department where he had a brilliant career until retirement. Today, he and his wife have two children, Danielle and Richard, and they in turn are married and have children of their own. They all live in England.

As far back as I can remember our family always had dogs—Scotties, West Highland Whites, and Dalmatians. On Christmas Eve of 1940, dad gave mom a six-week old gray female Dandie Dinmont Terrier.

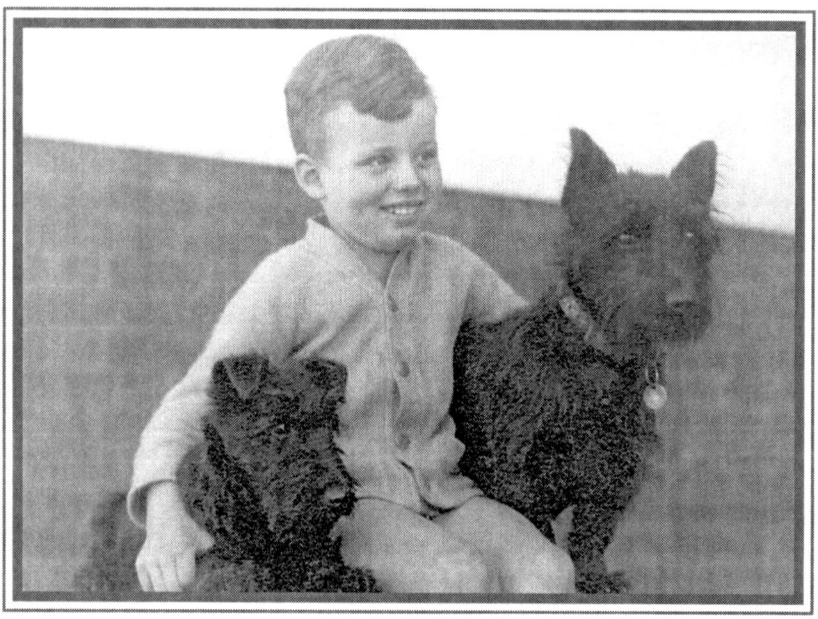

Ian and Scotties

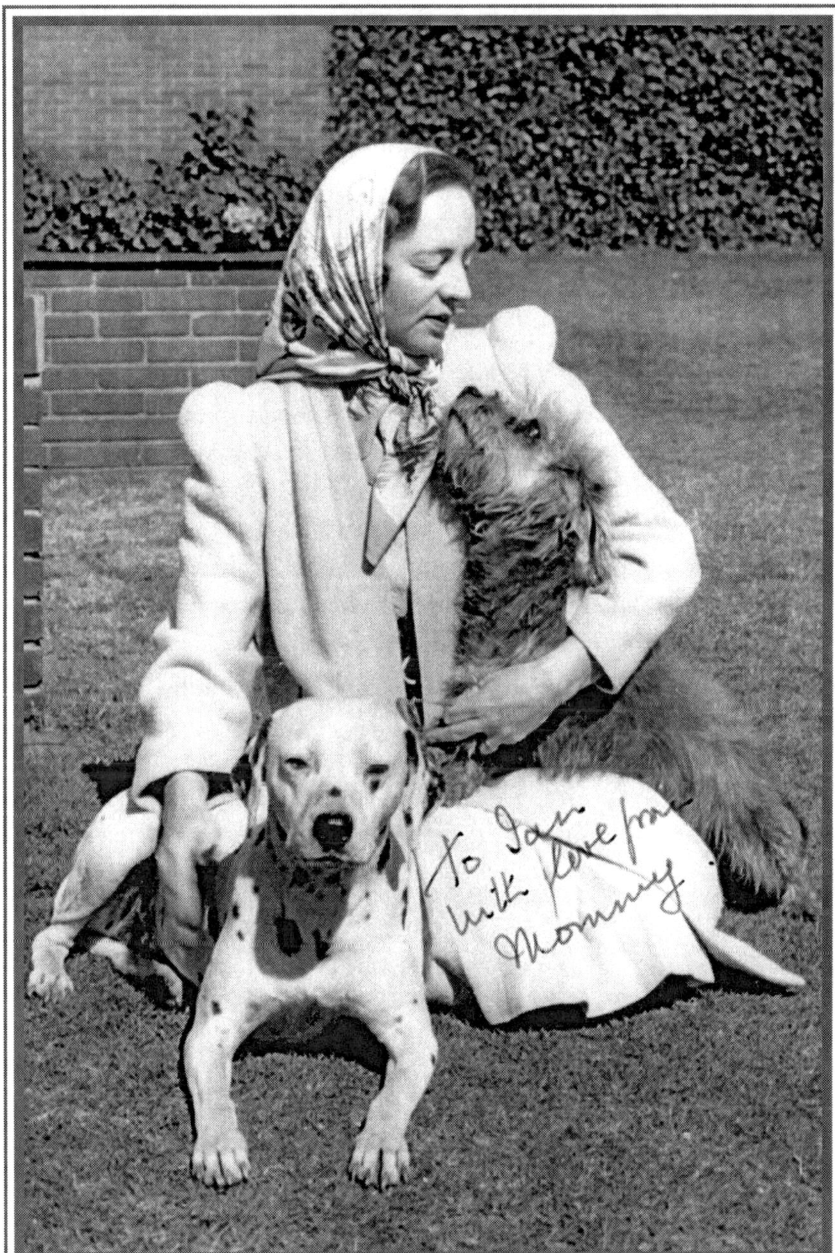

Mother with Dandie and Rubella

We had never heard of this breed before, Heaven alone knows how my father found this one! She came from Greytown in northern Natal, and mom named her Dandie. Not a very inspired name for a dog that would turn out to be the most memorable and courageous dog I have ever known.

When she was about eighteen months old, Dandie decided that she would be the custodian of our vegetable garden. We had many different vegetables and fruits, papaya, lychees, corn, and an old grapevine that produced delicious sweet black grapes.

The vegetable garden sloped down from our back lawn and had an eight-foot fence—no barrier to monkeys, who could easily scale it and ruin the vegetables, particularly the corn and the papayas!

Thick virgin bush surrounded our home. Here some of the world's most deadly snakes could hide. The green and black mamba snake can kill in minutes unless anti-venom is immediately available.

Dandie took her job seriously and always positioned herself on the grassy embankment near the top end of the vegetable garden. From this vantage point, her eyes could scan the entire garden and immediately observe intruders.

On one particular day, a V-shaped formation of egrets flew across a cloudless blue sky heading toward the Durban Bluff. Nearby one could hear the mournful cry of the tragedy bird. My mother named it the "tragedy bird" because it was black and had a sad, funereal quality to its three-tone bird call.

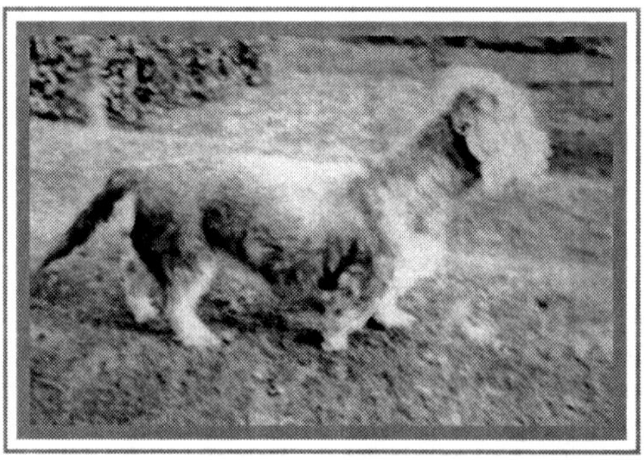
Dandie

Suddenly, an enormous monkey scaled the fence and climbed up a papaya tree. Dandie lay motionless, observing the monkey as it took random bites from a papaya. Her beautiful soulful eyes had transformed into those of an assassin as she readied herself for the kill.

The monkey was twice her size and had razor-like long nails. Dandie Dinmonts have extremely powerful backlegs and an amazingly strong lower jaw. As the monkey began to descend from the tree, Dandie sprang

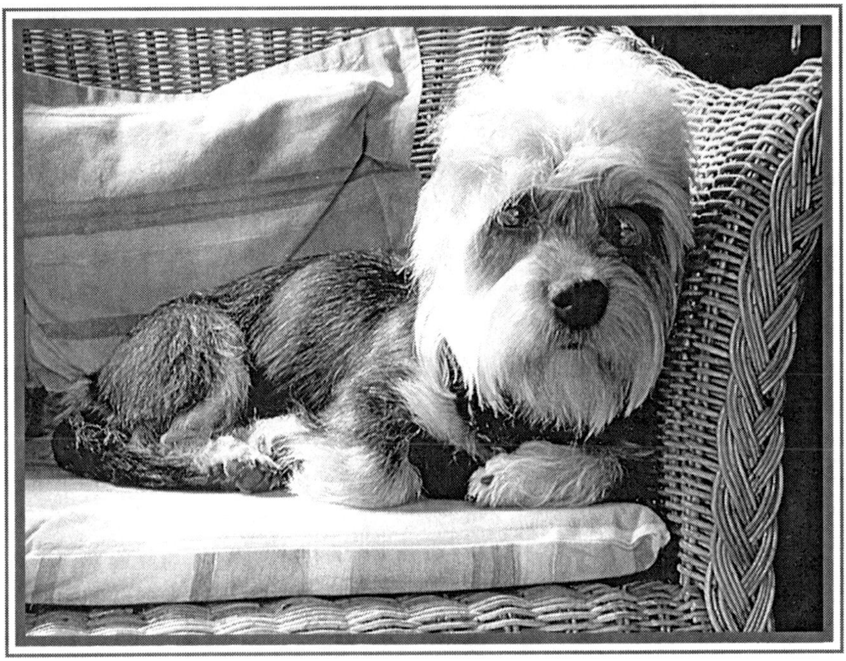

Wisdom

with lightning speed and remained waiting at the base of the papaya tree for the monkey to jump to the ground.

The monkey had not seen our self-appointed watchdog. It jumped to the ground and quickly stood up. In that split second, Dandie sprang for the monkey's throat, clamping down with her vice-like jaws and never relinquished her hold, until long after the monkey was dead.

John Mafeking witnessed the event. He was our one-handed garden "boy" (all of the male adult servants were called "boy"). John ran over to pull Dandie off the dead monkey.

The monkey's larynx was fractured and within minutes it lay lifeless, pieces of yellow papaya with its black seeds still on its mouth and face.

This encounter left Dandie with only a few very superficial scratches. Such had not always been the case, and on several certain other attacks we had to take her to the vet for stitches. In her lifetime, Dandie dispatched four of five monkeys to monkey heaven and proved to be a tremendous deterrent to the garden marauders.

As she became older, Dandie's reflexes slowed down and she developed cataracts. In a final encounter with an enormous monkey, Dandie was almost killed. She suffered serious lacerations, requiring sixty-seven stitches. This was the last time she sent a monkey to monkey heaven!

As the area we lived in began to develop for homes, the SPCA trapped the remaining monkeys and relocated them to a wildlife preserve—a much safer environment for them than our vegetable garden!

The last recollection I have of my mother's beloved Dandie, she was on the grassy embankment, her "look out." Her rheumy eyes were vigilantly looking for monkeys that would never return. I approached her slowly, sadly, as I had come to say goodbye. Dandie saw me coming. She gently wagged her tail and rolled over onto her back, showing me the enormous scar on her tummy that had required all those stitches. To this very day, whenever I think of our last goodbye I want to cry!

In my lifetime, I had four more dandies, but none could ever compare with the little gray bundle of fur my father brought home on December 24, 1940.

(This breed came in First in 2007 in the Terrier class at the Westminster Dog Show. The winner's name was Harry, and what a little champion he was!)

North Beach in Durban is a pristine, lovely beach with white sand firmly packed so one could easily walk for miles. The water was warm, and ideal for swimming and surfing. No wet suits necessary.

My parents often took me to North Beach on Sundays. During the winter month of July, a school holiday month, the beach was always crowded with people from Johannesburg, the Belgian Congo, and many other places.

The beachfront had several five-star hotels, our favorite being the Maharanee Hotel with deluxe rooms, all with balconies overlooking the Indian Ocean. Turbaned Indian waiters served scrumptious meals in the restaurants. Buffets of curried dishes ranged from very mild to incredibly hot, with at least "ten boys" to garnish the meal.

The term "ten boys" meant the number of bowls containing chutney, raisins, coconut, bananas, etc. When Britain ruled India, each bowl was carried by a single server. A young waiter, frequently referred to as "boy"—a somewhat derogatory term—carried each bowl.

(Many years later, my wife, Rosemary, and I were dinner guests of our friend, Martin, at his exclusive golf club in Montreal. Martin was a black Jamaican anesthesiologist. After having had an excellent meal, I enthusiastically said to our host, "Boy, that was a fine meal." Martin playfully responded, "Thank you, Master! ")

North Beach was packed as usual one Sunday when I first noticed two attractive young women sunning themselves. They were from the Belgian Congo, and I had remembered them from the previous year.

These women grew up in Europe, and were singularly devoid of inhibitions. Off came their tops, revealing beautiful tanned breasts as they applied suntan oil all over their bodies. What eye candy for a 13-year-old boy!

To gain an unobstructed view but not appear too obvious, I positioned myself behind two sunbathers sitting in deck chairs, about six feet from these lovelies. Lying on my stomach behind their chairs, I had a good view of the women—though I had to endure sand in my face kicked by the "deck chair sitters" whenever they wiggled their toes. It was worth it!

My physiological reaction to the view of these lovely semi-nude women was fast and furious. I was compelled to drape a beach towel around my middle every so often to cool off in the waters of the ocean, and then return shamelessly to my erotic pastime behind the beach chairs!

Lying at my usual vantage point, one lazy Sunday, I heard a terrible scream coming from the water—the horrified cry of a lifeguard being attacked by a shark! Although he was only in thigh deep water, a huge shark had struck without warning.

People on the beach began to run to the aid of the lifeguard and managed to drag him out from the bloody water. The shark had already virtually amputated his left leg. There was blood everywhere.

A well-known Durban plastic surgeon—an enormous man and close friend of my parents—Wally Visser (Colin's dad) was on the beach at the time. He placed his towel over the poor lad's gaping wound and applied intense pressure, probably saving his life since hemorrhage is the main cause of death from a shark bite.

An ambulance soon arrived and the ashen lifeguard was quickly transported to Addington Hospital, a short ride away. Father worked at Addington Hospital and was on duty that day, as was Mr. Percy Reardon, a skilled general surgeon. Dad administered the anesthetic and Mr. Reardon performed surgery. (Surgeons were addressed as "Mr." in the Commonwealth and England.) Despite multiple blood transfusions, the leg could not be saved.

Because of an increasing number of shark attacks, the municipality of Durban put out a shark net which stretched some hundred yards in length and fifty yards out from the shoreline. It was a straight net, open at each end. The rationale was that since sharks tend to swim in circles, many would be caught up in the nets. It worked, and greatly reduced shark attacks off Durban beaches.

My father was a workaholic, but the family still managed to take periodic holidays.

One such holiday was a visit to Victoria Falls, a four-day train ride away. We stayed at the Victoria Falls Hotel, a famous old hotel with a good dining room and an excellent bar. The name of the bar was "I Presume," named after Stanley and Livingston's famous meeting, "I presume."

There were frequent power failures at Victoria Falls, and we were given candles for illumination at the old firetrap hotel. Not very safe, but it worked.

I recall the menu in the dining room which featured crocodile meat. The caption of the menu read, "Eat the crocodile before it eats you." Crocodile and rattlesnake both taste very much like chicken.

The Victoria Falls are considered one of the Seven Wonders of the World. I can see why. The smoke that thunders (Mosi-Oa-Tunya) defies description. My parents and I took a plane ride in a single engine right over the mighty Falls one day, flying through a beautiful rainbow and capturing it on a 16mm kodachrome. Flying is undoubtedly the best way to see the Falls, to fully grasp the full grandeur.

Sad to say, our plane pilot, who routinely flew the Falls tours, lost his life years later in a crash into the Falls. Yet, perhaps that would have been his choice, if he had to go.

A delightful holiday was one up the Natal's north coast to a place called St. Lucia. Here one found flamingos by the thousands, crocodiles and hippos, a wildlife sanctuary and estuary.

Dr. Llewellyn Thomas was a friend of my parents. He was a little Welsh ENT specialist who smoked Gold Flakes cigarettes kept in a yellow tin. He loved Scotch whiskey, and had perpetual whiskey breath.

Dr. Llewellyn would often accompany us on some of our family holidays, since his wife did not like to travel. He and Dad were great storytellers, and they always had a good audience in me as I loved to listen to them.

On our visit to Victoria Falls, Dr. Llewellyn was with us. We rented an outboard motor boat one day, and the four of us set off for a day's outing. Nearby, an enormous crocodile was basking in the sun on a bank of the Zambezi River. Wanting to get a closer look and a shot with our movie camera, we moved in closer. Not a very smart thing to do.

As we came to within thirty feet of the prehistoric reptile, with small birds sitting on its back and its partly open mouth showing some vicious-looking teeth, our outboard motor suddenly konked out! Our little boat began to slowly drift toward shore as dad tried frantically to start the motor—to no avail.

The crocodile suddenly awoke from its snooze, opened an eye, and spotted us. In a flash, it dove under our boat and swam away. The boat rocked furiously, but did not capsize. Tommy Thomas came close to falling overboard as he attempted to catch the action on his 16mm movie camera. In the end, we were all disappointed when the film was developed and showed only Tommy's blurred white knuckles and no crocodile.

Well, we all had a good laugh over the crocodile incident—safely at home later in the day, that is. But I noticed many scotch whiskies were being consumed that evening. The most popular scotch in those days was "Dimple Haig," so named as the bottle had characteristic indentations resembling dimples.

"Don't be Vague, ask for Haig."

Hitler's armies attacked Poland on August 31, 1939, and on September 3, England and France declared war on Germany. I had just turned nine years old.

Father and his two younger brothers immediately signed up, but father was very disappointed when his application to enlist in the armed forces' medical core was rejected. He was needed to attend to the civilian population of Durban, he was told, since he was the most senior anesthesiologist in the country.

There was much excitement at home as my uncles proudly showed off their brand new uniforms, with hats propped jauntily on their heads. Both younger brothers went off to fight Field Marshal Erwin Rommel in North Africa in what was to be some of the bloodiest fighting in the Second World War.

Let me mention that the Afrikaner had no particular love for the English, and many were German sympathizers. A radical group of Afrikaners were members of a secret organization called the "Ossewabrandwag." They actively attempted to prevent South Africa from entering the war. However, our internationally famous Prime Minister of South Africa, General Jan Christian Smuts, managed to put a decisive stop to that.

I was a student at Clifton, my junior school, during the earlier war years. Klaus and Hubert were also students, twin brothers whose German father, Conrad Hertz, was a prominent Durban veterinarian. Dr. Hertz was caught red-handed transmitting information to German Intelligence in Lourenzo Marques, a coastal city in Portuguese East Africa (a neutral country).

The incident took place on an early morning in July of 1941. A special branch of the South African police force led by Captain Bertie Blaise-Smith and 2nd Lt. Koos Vandermerve, along with twelve heavily armed African police, converged on the small, insignificant looking rondaval not far from Botha's Hill. It was a hideout near Durban, on a promontory of land overlooking the Indian Ocean. At 4:00 a.m., the special unit crashed through the door of the rondaval and arrested Dr. Hertz in the act of traitorous espionage.

The information transmitted, gave detailed positions of ship convoys to the captains of German U-boats not far off the Natal coast. Unescorted troop carriers were easy prey, and many allied ships sunk as a result of such occult German U-boat activity.

Dr. Hertz spent the balance of the war in an internment camp. His two sons left Clifton, and I never saw them again.

Many British boys were evacuated from England to South Africa by their parents to escape the intense bombing. One of these was Henry, who became a classmate of mine at Clifton. Henry had red hair and freckles, and could whistle beautifully. His favorite tune was "Nola." If you're not from the Second World War era, you may not remember this tune!

Durban is a maritime city, and its port was of strategic importance for the passage of troops to the Far East, North Africa, and elsewhere. I remember well the Australian troops who visited Durban. A truly wild bunch! After a few South African Castle lagers, the Aussies once put a Rickshaw Boy into his own rickshaw and pulled him through the streets of Durban wearing his elaborate headgear. You should have seen the expression on the Rickshaw Boy's face!

There were frequent troop marches past our home on King George V Avenue. The troops looked so young, and many of them would be killed in action. What a terrible waste!

Durban turned out in force to welcome and entertain the troops. The Cosmo Nightclub did a roaring business with officers and Durban girls, all of whom had a whale of a good time. No doubt a "Tommy or two" would be left behind.

In truth, the Second World War seemed very remote to me as a young boy. South Africa was sofar away from the fighting. I had a map of France and drew the Maginot Line (the French line of resistance) and the Siegfried Line (the German one). In the early stages of the war, I marked the progress of the fighting with union jacks or swastikas pinned to the map.

There was a popular song in the early days of war in France—"We are going to hang our washing on the Siegfried Line." Famous last words.

The Germans completely outmaneuvered the French, and France fell in a very short space of time.

Dad had a shortwave radio, and we occasionally listened to shortwave broadcasts from Germany by Lord Haw-Haw. William Joyce was "Lord Haw-Haw," an American-born citizen raised in Ireland. He was the main broadcaster in English during the war, and he became a German citizen.

William Joyce had a "haw-haw" (hoity-toity) accent, and told the world how nicely Germany was doing—very well-orchestrated propaganda. Shortly before the end of the war, Joyce was captured by the English. He was tried and hanged for treason on January 3, 1946.

The war was still on when I entered high school at Michaelhouse. I realized with shock that some of the school's old boys were dying each week. Their names were read out on Sunday night at the end of the Chapel. The list grew longer and longer, and while I did not know any of the chaps it was sad to hear their names read from that list of those killed in action. Such is the legacy of war.

Our first home in Durban was a small, insignificant looking place at 80 Edmunds Road. As dad became more successful in his work, we moved to a more modern home. It was custom designed "art déco" in a bright yellow with a flat roof—ideal for sunbathing. The caption on the deck read, "Sun worshippers are we all." Such a complete contrast to the surrounding homes, but my parents loved it.

Dad named the home "Bradlaugh" after Sir Charles Bradlaugh, an English member of Parliament who made it possible to "attesting" as opposed to "swearing" on the Holy Bible in a court of law.

Dad was a member of the Rationalist Free Press Association, an organization that believed in the "supremacy of reason."

By 1940, we had moved to our third and final home, a mac-mansion high up on the Berea (Durban's hilly surrounding areas), on two acres of land. My parents paid 7000 British pounds for the home and

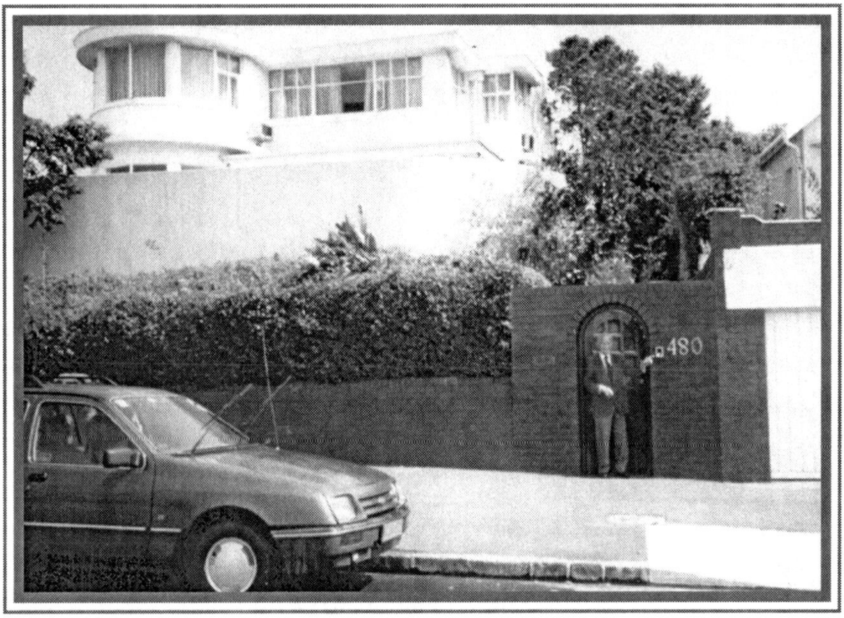

Bradlaugh

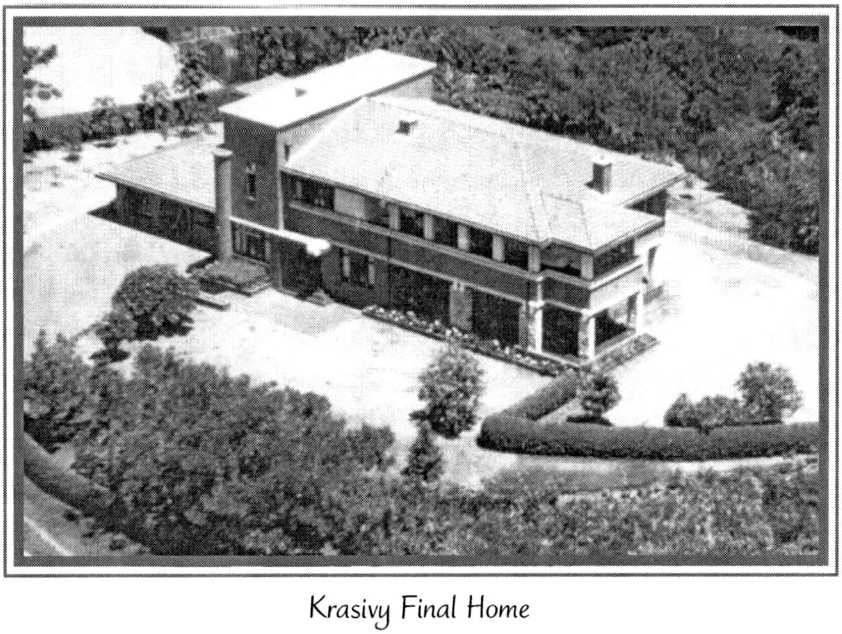

Krasivy Final Home

property, which was a lot of money in those days. It had a commanding view over the city of Durban, straight down Smith Street, West Street, and Durban's natural and beautiful harbor.

A white lighthouse stood on elevated ground (the bluff) near the harbor entrance. Tankers from all over the world could be seen waiting to gain entrance to the harbor.

Up on the sundeck of our house we had a spectacular 360-degree view northwards to the Valley of a Thousand Hills.

The surrounding virgin bush directly in front of our home was a natural wildlife preserve called Pidgeon Valley. It would one day be the ultimate tranquil resting place for the ashes of my grandmother, my mother, and my father.

My father became a wealthy man, not only through hard work but also through investments. He practiced medicine in an era when people loved, respected, and trusted their doctor.

Some of dad's patients were stockbrokers and accountants, and they would pass on priceless information to dad such as where the real "big boys" were investing their money (DeBeers, et al). These patients invested dad's money wisely, and just as he trusted them with his money, they trusted him with the health care of their families.

Harry Stevenson was one of dad's patients. He and a group of others were prospecting for gold one day near the Johannesburg Reef (the gold mining area). It was very hot that day and they had been walking for a considerable time. Harry's feet were sore so he stayed behind to cool off in a little nearby rivulet, and the group continued on without him. The water was clear and soothing, and as he soaked and wiggled his toes, Harry noticed a gold vein protruding in the water. Talk about landing on your feet! Harry had struck gold, big time!

The Stevenson Mine, as it was later called, was probably the largest producer of gold on the Johannesburg Reef. Dad was also a recipient of a share or two (or was it three?) in the Stevenson Mine, when gold was pegged at only thirty-five dollars an ounce.

Harold once gave dad a beautiful gold pocket watch inscribed, "To my dear and trusted friend Harry, (from) Harold R. Stevenson." I eventually inherited this watch, and one day I passed it on to our South African accountant, Jack, as a small token of appreciation for all the work he had done for us over the years.

Dad loved convertible Pontiacs and every few years would trade cars. One day, he brought home a brand new, fire engine red convertible. A beauty. He left it parked on our sloping driveway and, captivated and curious, I climbed into the front seat and released the hand brake.

The car began to slowly slide backwards, gathering speed on the incline as it crossed the road. It tore up a few bushes, and then smashed into an electric light pole! Nobody was hurt, and I was not reprimanded (thanks to the permissive school of child rearing, advocated by A.S. Neil). But dear old dad must have wept a tear or two in private!

On the subject of cars, Mr. Percy Reardon, a close friend of dad's, was one of Durban's foremost general surgeons. Mr. Reardon once ordered a Rolls-Royce from England. The expensive car arrived in South Africa nine months later! It would not start. It simply would not start, though Mr. Reardon tried everything. Since Durban did not have a Rolls-Royce dealership, the frustrated Mr. Reardon was finally obliged to contact the dealership in England, who sent a mechanic all the way to South Africa to service the automobile.

The mechanic began his diagnostics by feeling under the dashboard and turning a switch (security device). The car started like a dream!

Dad and Mr. Reardon often worked together, with dad administering the anesthesia for the surgery. Dad carefully examined a patient well before surgery. He administered the exact amount of anesthesia in order to allow the surgeon to work on a fully relaxed patient, and still permit the patient to wake up shortly thereafter.

Before departing the hospital, dad always made certain the patient's vital signs were stable. He would return later in the day to do a post-operative visit when the patient was fully awake. In those days, dad had to lug his own heavy anesthesia equipment in his car from hospital to hospital.

Dad was a real pro, but the fees for such expertise were roughly one-tenth of that charged by a surgeon. Today, both surgeon and anesthesiologist are compensated very much the same. And rightfully so!

My photograph albums are filled with snaps of the smiling faces of Africans. Over the years, we had many servants, and all deserve the very highest praise. Many of these wonderful people gave their whole lives to serving our family. In retrospect, we regarded this servitude as our God-given right.

The servants were all Zulus except for one Indian. The name given to them was "kaffir," which means "infidel." This is now an unacceptable name in South Africa.

The servants always managed to smile, and often sang their melodic, repetitive Zulu songs, with the rhythms coming from deep within their souls. I can still hear the music and see their lovely faces as clearly as if it were today.

My eyes easily blur with tears when I think of our servants. They were, after all, part of our family and we did love them. Yet, they had so little and we had so much—they deserved so much more from life.

There were separate rooms for the male and female servants, and they slept on bunk beds. The diet of the African seemed boring—a dish resembling porridge, which was called "putu." But they never seemed to tire of it.

Zulu is a beautiful language and the Zulus always speak with a certain softness. "Kunjani nKosana?" ("How are you, Master?") "Hamba Kahle, Sala Kahle." ("Go safely, stay safely.")

Though my family loved our servants, we really knew so little about them. How many wives and children did they have? How many cows? (Cows were a most important commodity because it was with cows that an individual could "purchase" a wife with labola (a type of dowry.) Where exactly did they come from in Zululand? They were separated from their families for months on end. Their income was appallingly low, and most of it was sent home to support their families.

As long as the servants did all the housework, cooked the meals, made the beds, cleaned our shoes, and did the gardening, we were satisfied. As long as they did not make too much noise putting away the dishes, and did not get too drunk on "kaffir beer" or a potent alcohol mix, umgombothi (Shimiaan), we were happy. This sad state of affairs was common among the whites, who regarded their master-servant relationships as sacrosanct.

Japtha served us most of his life. He came to us as a teenager, and today is an old man with gray hair. I recall how he loved to play football, and could have well represented South Africa in this sport had it not been for Apartheid.

A nasty disease once afflicted Japtha, and he turned to my mother who was a nurse and someone he trusted. She took him to a black hospital, King Edward VIII, for treatment, and our family paid his bill. When my father died in 1991, he left Japtha some well-deserved money. In these respects, we did show our love for the servants.

I had occasion to visit King Edward VIII Hospital many years later, an enormous general hospital catering to the black population. The maternity section was so overcrowded that some women in labor had to lie on the floor under the elevated beds.

Most women delivered at home or by the roadside in a squatting position. In many cases, local witch doctors would tie off the umbilical cord, rubbing cow dung into the infant's still-bleeding umbilicus. Cow dung contains tetanus bacilli, and would easily infect the newborn babies.

To witness tetanus neonatorum (tetanus of the newborn) was terribly sad. The convulsing infants lay side by side in hospital in a coffin-like structure, suffering and simply waiting to die.

Mother really could not boil water without literally burning it, so father acquired a cook and houseboy by the name of Cornelius. Cornelius came to us as a little boy and remained with us his entire life—a period of over forty years! His family lived in Zululand, and periodically Cornelius would be given time off for a visit to his family. Although Cornelius died before my father did, his family received a generous amount of money in my father's will.

Cornelius was a rotund, short man, with very little facial hair. He was soft-spoken, loyal, a hard worker—truly a delightful individual. He could also make the most wonderful fluffy omelets. We called them "Cornelius Specials." Many other of our servants could also be described as loyal and hardworking. John Ingelo was our first houseboy at 80 Edmunds Road, and a dear little man. He could not have been much more than five ft. four inches, was painfully thin, and blind in one eye. John did just about everything for our family, inside and outside, and was with us for many years.

Nookwa Zama, another servant, was a big, strapping fellow with very light skin. He had a short fuse, and I am quite certain I often irritated him with my undisciplined ways. There was an arrogant independence about Nookwa not seen in our other servants.

Our gardener, John Mafeking, had lost his hand in an industrial accident. The remarkable thing about John is that he could do more with his one hand than many people could do with two.

Dad had a rather serious accident in later years. Nobody was hurt, but his driving license was suspended. Thus, Simon entered our lives as dad's new chauffeur. Let's face it—there are worse things in life than having one's own chauffeur!

By no means could I ever forget our other Indian chauffeur, Gannas. Gannas was in his early twenties when he came to work for our family. He was tall and good-looking, always dressed well, and spoke beautiful English with no trace of an Indian accent. He was truly a prince of a man and the only person in my early life who gave me any—ouch! —discipline! When Gannas said "No," he meant "No."

Since Clifton School was quite far from home, Gannas drove me to and from school in our big black Packard. He taught me many things that were fun, such as how to make paper kites using sticky rice to glue the brown paper. I remember also how Gannas could iron beautifully. He was to stay with us for many years.

Gannas later invited our family to his wedding where we met his delightful bride in her beautiful blue and gold Sari. It was obvious how much in love they were. It was a fascinating ceremony—an Indian wedding I will never forget. The food alone was out of this world. It was a feast to remember, but mostly I recall the many curry dishes ranging from mild to extremely hot (mother-in-law) to even hotter (atomic) samosas.

Many years later on a visit to Durban to see my parents, I rang Gannas whom I had not seen in over fifteen years. My wife, Rosemary, and I wanted to visit with him.

At the time, apartheid was the law of the land (an official policy of racial segregation practiced in South Africa) and Gannas lived with his family in an Indian district, under this law. Many white people in South Africa were strongly opposed to Apartheid. Nonetheless, I had to gain permission from the police for our visit to see Gannas.

They lived in a simple home. Gannas was still handsome, and much grayer. We hugged and we cried. My old friend Gannas was still very special to me!

During dinner with Gannas and his relatives, Rosemary and I noticed that the other guests were all male. "Why does your wife not come and eat with us?" Rosemary asked. Gannas explained that his wife ate with her fingers—not an uncommon practice in some parts of the world—and she felt this might make us uncomfortable, so she dined alone in the kitchen.

An organization in South Africa founded in 1955 by Jean Sinclair was called The Black Sash. It was a nonviolent white women's resistance organization, and its members used the relative safety of their privileged racial classification to speak out against the erosion of human rights in their country. The striking black sashes were worn as a mark of mourning and to protest against a series of unjust laws.

The South African government was petrified of communism, and if there was the slightest suspicion of anyone being a communist or even a communist sympathizer, he or she could be put into prison for 180 days with no recourse to a lawyer.

My father's library contained several books on socialism and my mother, who was legitimately frightened of all this, decided to have those books burned! One such book was written by the "Red Dean" of

Canterbury, entitled "The Socialist Sixth of the World." It was a red book with a picture of a hammer and sickle on the front cover.

Dad later became involved in an organization during the Second World War called "Medical Aid for Russia," and he grew a Lenin-like goatee! Much to my mother's disapproval, I might add.

Dad and I once took "conversational Russian" lessons from a Mrs. Beecham. Russian is not a particularly easy language! After the war ended, dad went to Russia on several occasions to visit Russian hospitals in his line of work. The staff there had never heard Russian spoken with a South African accent!

In 1945, I entered Michaelhouse, an all-boys private school located about thirty minutes north of Pietermaritzburg, the capital of Natal, and one of South Africa's four provinces. The school was well over a hundred years old, situated 3000 feet above sea level in a most beautiful part of Natal with rich rolling hills and breathtaking scenery.

Natal is so steeped in history as to merit some mention. It was the site of some of the bloodiest of Zulu wars. The battle of Blood River, for example, took place on December 16, 1838 when the Boer, Andries Pretorius's 470 determined Voor trekkers, defeated 10,000 Zulu on the banks of Ncome River. Today, December 16 is a public holiday in South Africa called "Dingane's Day."

Zululand has had many Zulu chiefs—Dinuzulu, Cetshwayo, Dingane, to name a few. One chief stands out far above all others—Chaka, Zulu king and warrior (1786-1828). In the ten years he ruled the Zulu nation, there were over two million deaths from warfare attributed to Chaka. There were also countless others who died trying to escape his ruthless armies.

The famous Chaka's Rock overlooking the Indian Ocean on Natal's North Coast Road is the site of where, rumor has it, Chaka and his buddies threw unlucky prisoners to certain death. Infants deformed at birth suffered a similar fate. An early example of active euthanasia!

Whenever I visit the Valley of a Thousand Hills, I imagine I can hear the echo of Chaka's Zulu warriors chanting, "Hold him down, you

Zulu warrior, Zulu warrior, Zulu warrior. Hold him down, you Zulu chief, Zulu chief, chief, chief . . . " as the echoes gradually fade away into the distant hills.

Mangosuthu Chief Buthelezi is the leader today of the Zulu Nation. Shortly after Nelson Mandela's release from prison in 1990, Ted Koppel interviewed Mandela on ABC's "Nightline." People telephoned in from all over the world, congratulating Mandela on his release after twenty-seven years in prison on the infamous Robben Island.

Chief Buthelezi also phoned in from South Africa and asked Mandela why he had not heard from him since his release. Mandela replied, "I don't want to wash our dirty linen in public." It was an interesting remark, perhaps suggesting that Mandela may have unintentionally revealed some sort of tribal rivalry? There are many different dialects and languages among the tribes of South Africa, and thus inherent potential tribal problems exist.

I had never been away from home for any length of time, so I was apprehensive on my first day at Michaelhouse High School in Natal. Being a young new boy in a strange environment can be very intimidating.

The impressive ivy-covered main building of Michaelhouse and its chapel with beautiful stained glass windows can be seen from the approaching road. Lush green playing fields for cricket and rugby, the main sports, surround the buildings. Tennis courts, squash courts, and a large swimming pool make for a real sportsman's paradise!

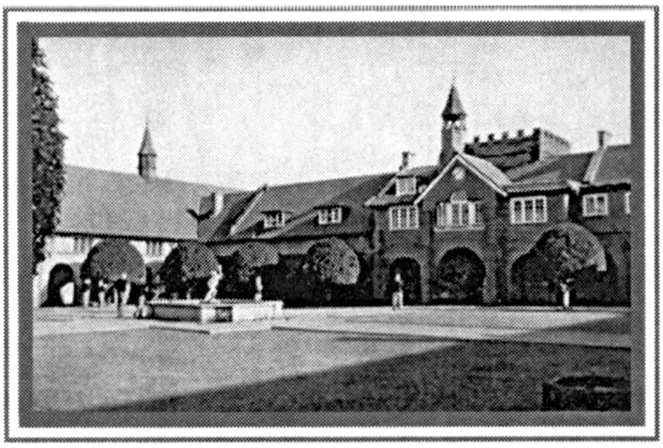

Michaelhouse (1945-1947)

The school deified sports, as I did, and I soon became athletic captain of East House. My best time in the half-mile was two minutes and seven seconds—not too far off a school record!

Michaelhouse had a snobby reputation, under normal circumstances, but when a certain rugby player on our team once shouted, while scrumming (rugby term) against a rival team, "A little more pressure in the rear, boys! " (What should have been said, was, "Push like hell, you lazy bastards! ")

Michaelhouse never quite lived down the expression, "A little more pressure in the rear, boys!" confirming the snobby reputation forever.

The entrance at Michaelhouse leads into a large quadrangle with dormitories, classrooms, a dining hall, and a library. I settled in well, and the next three years would be some of the happiest of my life.

Modeled on the British public school system, Michaelhouse is far from being public. The tuition is expensive. Boys came from well-to-do families, some with old money and some with new. There were no black students when I was there (from 1945 to 1947), but this would change in time.

Education at Michaelhouse was excellent. Many of the masters (teachers) came from universities, such as Oxford or Cambridge. Michaelhouse students themselves often went on to those esteemed universities.

My ultimate goal was to enter Cambridge University Medical School in England, but I sometimes worried that it might be easier for a dyslexic to gain entry into heaven than Cambridge. There were so many brilliant applicants from all over the world, I was not sure I had a fighting chance. In recent survey of world universities, Cambridge University ranked number two, second only to Harvard.

School days soon passed much too quickly. Strict discipline and rules were enforced from the beginning, and new experiences came to me often in my home away from home.

Surprisingly, winter weather was very cold. Not accustomed to such weather, I managed to get a severe case of chilblains during my first winter. Chilblains are a frostbite-like condition of the fingers and toes—bloody painful, and hardly the thing one expected in a place like sunny South Africa!

There were eight houses at Michaelhouse, each with its own name.

Every student was assigned to one of these houses and my assignment was to Foundation East. Wilber Smith, a year or two my junior, was assigned to Founders House. The houses were large communal dormitories with bathing facilities, and each had its own housemaster (senior schoolteacher) and prefect (a position of distinction conferred on a few final-year students).

Daily life was strictly regimented. Six a.m. wake-up with hot tea or chocolate and very hard rusks (rock-hard objects that had to be dipped in whatever you were drinking).

A cold plunge or shower would take care of most recalcitrant early morning erections! New boys, known as "cacks," had various tasks to perform, as well—for example, cleaning the prefect's shoes, or sitting on the freezing cold toilet seats to warm them up for seniors. A most degrading task.

Meals were served in a large dining hall where we ate at long benches. The "House head prefects" trooped into the dining room to sit together at a separate table and take turns saying grace at the beginning of each meal. "Benedictus, Benedicat, praesum christum dominus nostrum."

The food was terrible, and I sorely missed Cornelius's cooking. We new students, all somewhat pampered blokes, immediately balked at what we called "penis" butter sandwiches and "Granny's tits" (stewed prunes).

To make matters worse, giant-sized oil paintings of previous rectors ("rectums") hung on the wood-paneled walls, staring down at us disapprovingly during mealtime mayhem.

Classes took place before breakfast and again before lunch, followed by several hours of sporting activities. There was homework after dinner, followed by lights-out at 10:00 p.m.

Soon after lights-out, the Vaseline jars surreptitiously appeared, followed by suppressed cries of masturbating delight!

Thus ended a typical day, and all was quiet at Michaelhouse.

My first introduction to God soon arrived and I tried to become a good Christian by being confirmed, casting aside the last shreds of

Judaism. (There were only a few token Jewish boys besides me). Grace was said before meals, church was attended on Sundays, and communion was taken regularly.

I am ashamed to admit to an ulterior motive for my becoming confirmed. By going to early communion on Sundays, I could get out from school much earlier on our leisure "day of rest." We all looked forward to Sundays when we could hike in the picturesque countryside, or possibly hitch a ride to Durban, eighty miles away. Sometimes our parents came to visit with picnic baskets laden with delicious homemade food. Yes, we loved our Sundays.

My best friend at the time, Aubrey, was a polite, gentlemanly lad, and we had many good times together. We hitched a ride one Sunday from a couple heading to Durban from Johannesburg. They were driving a brand new 1945 Studebaker, an interesting looking car because one could not tell the front from the back! The driver drove like a maniac, possibly trying to compete with Sir Malcolm Campbell. Scared the bloody hell out of us.

(Sir Malcolm Campbell had established a world speed record on September 3, 1935 with his "Bluebird" by racing to 301 mph, or 481.81 kph)! I saw this incredible racing car several years later, when it came to Durban.)

Still on the subject of daredevils, I must mention Bradley who had attended Michaelhouse several years earlier. As the story goes, Bradley and a friend hitchhiked to Howick one Sunday, not far from Pietermaritzburg. The Howick Falls are 105 meters high, just a little lower than the Victoria Falls. On a dare, his friend said, "I'll bet you wouldn't dive over."

Bradley took the dare and, regrettably, Dare Devil Bradley became history.

My family's friend, Mr. Reardon (the Durban surgeon), had a beautiful country home within easy walking distance of Michaelhouse. He also had two beautiful daughters.

Italian prisoners of war had built Mr. Reardon's house. They were master craftsmen, especially skilled with their wrought ironwork. Many of these Italian prisoners stayed on after the war, and became very successful in the construction business.

One Sunday, while walking to the Reardon's country home to visit his daughters and scrounge lunch, I narrowly missed being struck by lightning. I saw the lightning strike the long grass very nearby, which swayed furiously and was accompanied by a sizzling sound. Instinctively, I dropped to the ground and was not struck. A most frightening experience.

Mr. Reardon had once been a medical student at Pembroke College Cambridge. He knew the senior tutor, a Mr. Laird Campbell. As time drew nearer for me to send in my application to Cambridge, Mr. Reardon wrote to Mr. Campbell, blowing my trumpet. (One goes Up to Cambridge and Down to London! If you are "sent down," that means goodbye to Cambridge—forever!)

In those days, the Old Boy Grapevine was alive and well, but one still had to come up with the marks!

A debating society met once a week in the library, and in my last year I became our team's captain. Debates against other schools included a girl's school, St. Agnes College. At one such debate, the topic of discussion concerned "crooning." "Are crooners good singers, or should they be abolished?"

I had the balls to stand up and croon the melody, "Sentimental Journey." Well! The girls literally swooned, and of course, our team won the debate! I found debating to be great fun, and our team seldom lost.

Ladies of St. Agnes School often attended the dances held at Michaelhouse. We were given program cards, and our approach was to come up to a young lady and say, "May I please have the pleasure of this dance?" All very formal.

Chaperones were always present at our dances to assure there was no hanky-panky. About the most any of us boys managed was to slip a surreptitious hand beneath a girl's blouse, and fumble. We called this "fraying."

Mr. Sean McDuff, our biology teacher, was one such chaperone. He was also a homosexual. Mr. McDuff sounded very much like he had just got off the boat from Scotland, and he had a problem with wheezing. (It was also reliably reported that McDuff had a large shock of curly black pubic hair and a very small penis!)

Sitting at our desks in biology classes, Mr. McDuff would often press against our buns, ostensibly to oversee our work. The hornier he got, the more we would wiggle our posteriors, and the louder Mr. McDuff would wheeze! We students thought this hilarious, and became experts at imitating his wheeze. McDuff never had a clue.

There were very few anti-Semitics at Michaelhouse, but one incident does come to mind. While downstairs in the locker room one day changing my shoes, Tike Steward came in and said, "What are you doing, Jew boy?"

I was very taken aback at this remark and replied, "Would you mind repeating that, sir?"

Tike was a nasty bit of work with a pig-like face and shifty eyes, two years older than me and at least twenty pounds heavier. (He was nicknamed "Tike" because he was a shit disturber, of the first order.)

Before Tike could say one word, I struck him full force with my left fist in his solar plexus. My ambidextrous skills kicked in, and with my right arm encircling his neck I threw him to the concrete floor. A judo instructor would have been proud of me.

Tike was completely surprised and off balance, and fell to the floor with a resounding whack. He did not move for some time, and for a moment I thought I might have killed the bastard! But he opened his eyes—still groggy, with a frightened look on his face. I said, "Tike, old chap, I do hope I didn't hurt your feelings! " Tike never messed with me again.

I don't want to brag, but I was very strong in those days and had lightning reflexes—probably as a result of dodging Mr. Lewin's chalk!

When World War Two ended in 1945, my friends and I built a big bonfire to celebrate. It was on a clear evening, and the sky was filled with stars. We sat around the bonfire that evening and sang out loud and lusty, one song after another. I can clearly see those shining schoolboy faces lit up in the glow of the bonfire.

"Give me land, lots of land, 'neath the starry skies above." Then, the ever popular, "Hold him down, you Zulu warrior; hold him down, you Zula chief, chief, chief, chief, chief."

"Lula, I love you, honey, love you in the springtime and the fall; honey, honey, honey. Last night I had a dream, the sweetest dream of all, and in that dream I heard a scream, and thought it was my honey, honey Lula." Next verse!

"Morphine Bill met Cocaine Sue, walking down Fifth Avenue; so honey, have a sniff, have a sniff on me; honey, have a sniff on me. They came to a signpost painted green; the signpost said, 'there's no morphine'—so honey, have a sniff, have a sniff on me; honey, have a sniff on me."

"Ash to ash and dust to dust, if cocaine doesn't get you, morphine must! In the graveyard on a hill, lies the body of Cocaine Bill; and in the graveyard by his side, lies the body of his morphine bride. So for the last time, honey, have a sniffffff, on me! "

The growing list of names at Sunday Chapel (announcing the old boys from Michaelhouse who were killed in action) suddenly stopped! The war was over.

In my final year at Michaelhouse, I frequently visited the library to memorize, by copying and pasting into my brain's photographic memory bank, the answers to the last ten years of matriculation questions. I did not realize what I was fortuitously doing—that is, computing with my brain's "Windows 36" long before the advent of computers.

It was interesting that I had no problem speaking, and could be most articulate, yet I had so much difficulty reading and writing. Today I know that this is characteristic of dyslexia.

Hard labor at school paid off. Failure was not an option because I knew how disappointed my father would be. All of my life I admired dad's industrious hard work and hard play. "Per Ardua ad Astra," he would say. "Through hard work, you will reach the stars."

After three years, I left Michaelhouse with high marks and a first-class matric, thanks entirely to my photographic memory! I was seventeen.

Aubrey, my best friend from Michaelhouse, invited me to his home the following Christmas. We stayed with his parents who owned a pig farm near Pretoria. What a bloody awful smell!

It was during this Christmas visit with Aubrey that I met his cousin, Cynthia, who immediately became my very first real girlfriend. I was in love.

Cynthia had a pretty, oval-shaped face, and gorgeous long legs. She was always smiling. A most passionate kisser! But what more can I say? Christmas was soon over, and that was the end of it—almost.

The following school year, both Cynthia and I attended Cape Town University as freshmen. There she jilted me for an older man, a senior. I was crushed, but not for long as I had a healthy eye for pretty girls—and there were many pretty girls at Cape Town University.

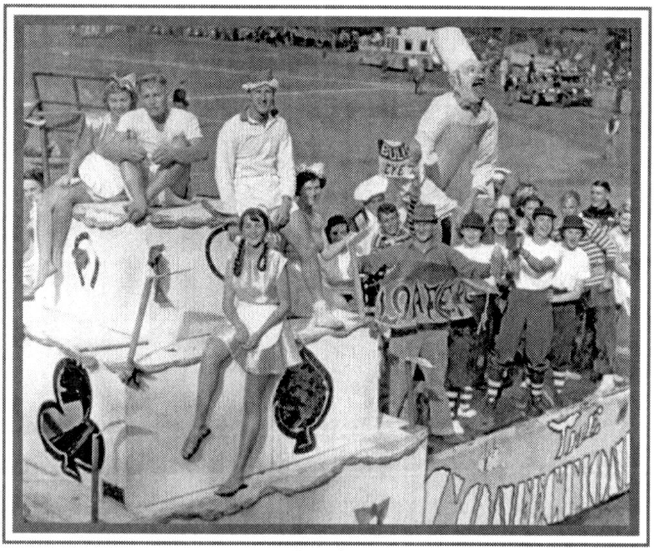

Cynthia

Before departing for Cape Town University, dad decided I should learn to drive a car. (Rule Number 1: Parents should never teach their children how to drive!) Dad gave me my first driving lesson, which lasted less than 15 minutes.

Since my dyslexia caused me to confuse left from right, pandemonium promptly ensued. Right off the bat, dad got angry and yelled at me. That was the end of it! (He later apologized, but decided it best to hire a "professional" instructor.)

My new instructor, a Mr. Fred Ainsley, was a skinny little bloke with slightly slurred speech, and his Harris tweed sports coat always reeked of tobacco. But he never yelled. Mr. Ainsley actually never got emotional about anything at all.

During the course of my "professional" driving lessons, riots were taking place in Durban. The year was 1949. The Zulus thought that the Indians were overcharging for bus fares—and they probably were! The Indians were shrewd business people and monopolized the Durban transportation.

The riots were becoming serious. Many Indian homes were being set on fire. Horrid rumors spread that Indian babies were being thrown into the fires! It was during this uproar that Mr. Ainsley and I inadvertently made our way into the rioting streets. I was at the wheel.

The commotion of the rioters was alarming. Bottles and stones went whistling past our windshield, but "No Worries Mr. Ainsley" just took a large swig of scotch from his half-jack and passed it over to me.

Some of the South African Indians actually did well for themselves in life as lawyers and doctors, having studied overseas for their degrees. They also became successful entrepreneurs in tailoring, dry cleaning, and marketing of fruit and vegetables. Many drove Rolls-Royces, and lived quite well.

Still, prejudice and "class distinction" often dies hard. I recall an incident when, in later years, I was admitted to a hospital in Durban as a patient. There were three of us in the coronary care unit. Besides me, there was an elderly Afrikaner woman in for observation and an Indian in his forties suffering from a coronary thrombosis.

The Afrikaner woman, Mevrou Van de Merwe, suddenly shouted in a loud voice, "What is this "coolie" doing in our ward?"

"Mevrou Van de Merwe, this young man has had a heart attack," I said. "If you go on insulting him, you may give the poor fellow another one, and he may possibly die! "

My reprimand to the Afrikaner woman went unheard. The Indian simply had no business being in a white ward!

During the six years in which my father was in general practice in Durban, one of his patients was a diabetic and very poor. Dad treated him, but never sent a bill.

Finally, after receiving good treatment for many months, the patient asked Dad why a bill was never submitted? The patient went on to explain that Alfred Hitchcock was his cousin, and paid all of his bills!

I trust dad commenced to send bills in a timely fashion to the "poor" patient.

One of the most beautiful cities in the world is Cape Town, surely on a par with the likes of Sydney, Vancouver, and Rio. The massive Table Mountain overlooks the city and harbor below, and a cable car runs to the top of the mountain where the views are spectacular. From there, one can look out to where the Indian and Atlantic Oceans meet at Land's End. When clouds envelop the top of Table Mountain (the "tablecloth"), cable cars do not run, and the magnificent panoramic views of Cape Town with its natural harbor and oceans become obscured.

Families of baboons hung out at Land's End. They often jumped on the hoods of automobiles, looking for a handout. With the arrival of new housing developments, the baboons' natural habitat slowly eroded and multiple baboon home invasions occurred!

Vineyards, wineries, and beautiful Old Dutch Colonial homes can be seen everywhere. Steeped in history, Cape Town is the place where early settlers made their home and called it the Cape of Good Hope. There were many shipwrecks in the rough and treacherous waters at Land's End as the early settlers attempted to round The Cape of Good Hope.

(As an unrelated "aside"—should you happen to be in possession of a South African black triangular penny stamp, you are the owner a small fortune! Check it out.)

The world famous "Blue Train" travels from Cape Town to Johannesburg and back. This overnight journey is spectacular and should not be missed by anyone on a visit to South Africa. The most picturesque part of this trip must surely be the lovely vineyards seen as one arrives or departs Cape Town. These vineyards produce some of the finest wine in the world. Train passengers enjoy five-star cuisine, fine wine, and impeccable service.

The backdrop of beautiful mountain ranges (while getting tipsy from all that wine!) indeed makes for a very special train experience.

In January of 1948, I entered the University of Cape Town as a premed student. To have arrived this far in my studies—despite severe dyslexia and my continued inability to read—was incredible, but all made possible by using my brain's "Windows 36! "

De Waal Drive is an excellent road leading to the UCT via a short ride from the center of Cape Town. Along this road, one passes University Hospital, Groote Schuur, where Dr. Christian Barnard performed the world's first heart transplant.

The university is located directly below Table Mountain. Graduation ceremonies take place at Jamieson Hall, which has a commanding view of the men's and women's residences and the athletic playing fields. The men's residence consisted of "flats," with about ten students per flat, each with his own bedroom.

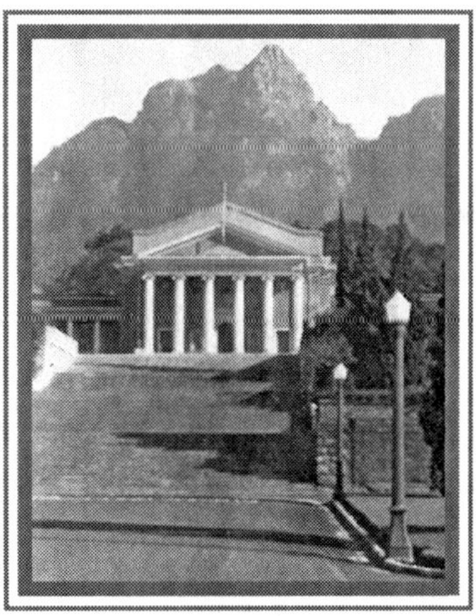

Jamieson Hall

Students at the university came from all over South Africa. Some were Afrikaners. Half were medical students, and the balance studied engineering, law, and architecture.

UCT freshmen (first year) students were subjected to one year of various initiation indignities—such as having to wear a twelve-inch green bow tie at all times. Quite degrading when one is trying to attract girls, and it cut down considerably on our dating prospects.

At UCT, I made some cherished friendships. Jerry Stein was one such friend, and we became close quickly. He came from a poor family, but nonetheless earned six "A's" on his matriculation! He was an excellent rugby player, and an incredibly hard worker. We often studied together evenings if we weren't out looking for girls.

As a first-year medical student, four subjects were required—Physics, Chemistry, Botany, and Zoology. If I hoped to gain entry to Cambridge University, I had to get high marks in all of these subjects.

There were 184 medical students, all with first-class matriculations, writing the first year final examinations. Only one hundred students succeeded in passing. I was in the magic one hundred! My photographic memory had saved me once again!

After hearing of the results, Jerry looked at me with great admiration (and surprise), and said, "I confess, I never thought you'd make it."

Jerry and I stayed in touch for many years. In my last Christmas card to him, I enclosed a snapshot taken of us together at "Men's Res" in 1948. Sad to say, Jerry's wife received my card one week after Jerry had died from inoperable cancer. My good friend was gone.

There were many such friends over the years, but it becomes difficult to stay in touch. Eventually the Christmas cards stop coming, and one begins to outlive old friends. After first year at Cape Town University, I remained for an additional six months to study anatomy and physiology, and to prepare for an organic chemistry exam which was a further requirement of Cambridge.

The memorable days at lovely Cape Town all too soon ended, and I returned to Durban for a brief stay before moving on to England. Back home, something was missing! Lizzie, our white servant, who had been with us for as long as I could remember, had been fired!

I was never able to find out the details, but I had a feeling there were some shenanigans by Lizzie with my younger brother, Peter. I imagine my mother may have walked in on something. Fare thee well, Lizzie, old girl, wherever you are.

I found myself remembering how my parents would yell at Lizzie or other servants for making noise with the dishes in the kitchen! Much later in time—when I myself had to wash and put away my own dishes—I realized that it is virtually impossible to put away dishes without making some noise!

I began to prepare for my move, and excitement ran high. The moment finally arrived. I was on my way to Cambridge to begin a life of incredible and superb experiences.

The move meant my final goodbye to South Africa. While I would visit often during the coming years, I would never again live in the beloved country where I was born.

If you want to imitate a South African accent, just clip your words (wurds), milk (mulk), kill a white (kila wat). And just speak like a ventriloquist! Got it?

After leaving South Africa, people often asked me where I came from. I cringed and mumbled a response, because South Africa was considered the polecat of the Southern Hemisphere.

In 1952, a law was enacted forcing South African blacks or colored people to carry a "pass card." The card contained a photograph and information about one's color and nationality, and it could be demanded by authorities at any time. Failure to have this pass card in one's possession could result in prison or relocation. Apartheid put racism into law. Nelson Mandela had such a card, but he burned it!

My wife, Rosemary, and I once met a couple who were traveling around the world. The man had a South African accent, which I recognized immediately, and we struck up a conversation. He told us the following distressing story:

This man grew up in Cape Town and was considered white. He looked as white as any white person—but he was colored. He had a black grandmother who lived in "District Six" in Cape Town. District Six was in many ways a unique community. There was a mixture of whites, blacks, coloreds, Christians, Muslims, Hindus, and other ethnic backgrounds—

all living together in harmony. The district was created as a suburb for lower income workers, and lies just west of Cape Town's downtown area.

When the man's father changed jobs his pass card was scrutinized and it was then discovered that he was not technically a white man at all. The usual consequences resulted.

In 1966, District Six was declared a "whites only" area and the community which had been there for generations was bulldozed into oblivion, including his grandmother's home.

To conclude my writings on South Africa, many people who lived there in the apartheid era loved the country as much as my family and I did. It is fair to say that we all enjoyed a peaceful lifestyle, one essentially laid back and safe.

Over the years, crime and violence have become rampant in South Africa. People are afraid, most of the time. They keep their windows and doors locked. Rape, murder, harassment, robbery, and terrorism—this is today's South Africa, and I hurt for it.

But an incident occurred which gave me hope for a happier future for sunny South Africa. As I was driving in Durban during a vacation from university, I came upon an accident. An elderly Zulu had been knocked off his bicycle, and his gray head was covered in blood. People had gathered around him, and I stopped to see if I could help. An ambulance was on its way.

With the butt of a gun sticking out from her jacket pocket, a white woman kneeled on the ground and cradled the head of the old black Zulu in her lap until help arrived.

With human kindness such as this, there is hope for a better future for South Africa.

England

- 1949 -

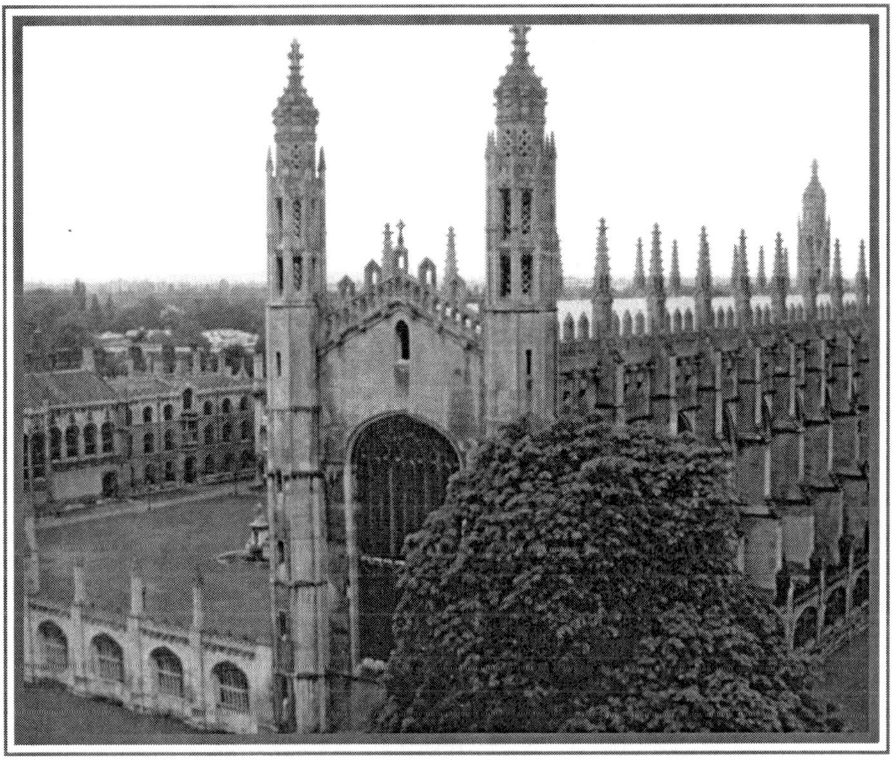

Kings College, Cambridge

On September 27, 1949, I occupied a plane seat on Royal Dutch Airline (KLM)—a man of the world, off to study medicine at Cambridge. You could say I was full of myself, bright-eyed and eager, standing on the threshold of adult life with wonderful opportunities ahead.

A Mr. Scott, Esq., Tommy Llewellyn Thomas's brother-in-law, occupied the seat next to me. He was a fine, elegant man (slightly pompous), and an English lawyer who many years later would be knighted and become England's Lord Chief Justice. Sitting together in the plane, I told him about my Christmas visit to Aubrey's family pig farm and my romance with Cynthia. "I'll bet the farm smelled like a Japanese wrestler's jockstrap," he said.

Mr. Scott would one day (in 1964) be the judge to sentence the great English train robbers to a collective three hundred years in prison. The story has it that thieves had ambushed the Glasgow to Euston mail train and pinched over two million pounds in unmarked bank notes in the biggest-ever raid on a British train!

The brilliantly planned operation involved twelve bank robbers. Charlie Wilson was captured in 1968 and Bruce Reynolds in 1969. Ronnie Biggs had escaped and remained free for nearly forty years!

When he was 71 years old (in 2001), Ronnie Biggs returned to Great Britain from Brazil where he had been living to receive free medical treatment after having suffered a series of strokes. Had he blown all that money? Ah, the luck of the Irish failed the notorious Mr. Biggs. Abruptly captured, he was sent to prison for twenty-eight years.

It was common practice in those days for judges to visit the prisons where they had sent malevolent blighters for crimes committed. Mr. Justice-Scott paid such a visit many years following the train robbery. He was standing in the prison's cafeteria lunch line that day, when he felt a tap on his shoulder. Turning around, he looked suddenly into the eyes of one of the train robbers.

"Just wait until we get out," warned the ill-fated and disgruntled robber. Famous last words.

Our plane landed safely in London and I was met by my old friend, Colin Visser (openly gay and a one-time member of the infamous

Elephant 8). Colin was studying in London at the Royal Academy of Dramatic Art.

Since I had some free days before reporting to Cambridge, Colin invited me to stay with him at his apartment at Karen's Gate Gardens for some outings. Without further ado, Colin took me to his favorite gay bar.

I was a straight young lad and interested only (but fervently) in girls, yet I watched with fascination as men danced together at the gay bar, hugging and kissing each other! I had never seen such goings-on. But it was nothing compared to the renowned Turkish Bath House I was to visit with Colin on a later outing. (I admit I did not accompany him half-heartedly. Quite the contrary, I was very curious.)

Inside the bathhouse, clouds of steam did not fully disguise the shenanigans taking place among the nude "bathers." Towels were quickly tossed. "Let the games begin with rim!"

Colin soon took up with a young man and disappeared somewhere into the steam. Left alone, I felt awkward and ill at ease. I clutched a towel around my middle and sat down to observe, with fascination, the muggy sex scene around me.

By and by, out of the thick haze a man approached me—naked as a Jay Bird—with all of his manly virtues prominently flaunted. He introduced himself as "Mike."

You can imagine, I was quite frozen with shock and sat very still, not making the slightest move. Jay Bird must have read this as "consent" on my part. He lay down close beside me with an erotic "come hither" smile on his face, slowly removed my towel, and began to give me a very personal massage!

I returned promptly to my wits, sprang to my feet, grabbed my towel, and made an insane dash for the locker room. As I deftly attempted to sidestep feet, rear-ends, and what-have-you, a few irritable obscenities were nonetheless yelled my way.

I was dressed and out the door before you could say "Jack Robinson." Another new record for Ian, I suspect.

There is something sacred and wonderful about walking the grounds of a great learning institution.

Cambridge University is such a place. When I first set foot on the grounds of Cambridge as a new medical student in 1949, the exhilaration of it all hit me like a ton of bricks. I could still not read, yet this prestigious university had accepted me, and I was here! It was a magic day for me.

Cambridge University's beautiful architecture alone was impressive, and King's College Chapel is the epitome of Gothic architecture. Its choir is world famous, with music to soothe and uplift the soul! I can hear still those beautiful young voices singing "Amazing Grace."

The ancient buildings date back to possibly the year 1209. Story has it that Cambridge University could trace its origins to a crime committed in 1209. Two Oxford students were hanged that year—with the consent of the King—for the murder of a woman. Dispute and outrage by Oxford students followed, and they commenced to migrate to Cambridge. Ever since, the universities of Oxford and Cambridge have retained a long history of rivalry between them.

Cambridge is the second oldest university in the English-speaking world and one of the most prestigious. There are currently thirty-one colleges within the University, of which three admit only women (New Hall, Newnam and Lucy Cavendish). Originally, only male students were accepted, but in 1869 Girton College was opened to women and Newnam College followed in 1872.

Historically, Cambridge has produced a significant proportion of the world's prominent scientists, writers, politicians, and others. To name a few: Sir Francis Bacon (Trinity College); Lord Byron (Trinity); Charles, Prince of Wales (Trinity); Charles Darwin (Christ's); Oliver Cromwell (Sidney Sussex); Ted Hughes (Pembroke); Isaac Newton (Trinity); Lord Alfred Tennyson (Trinity).

I must confess that, despite my acceptance to this great university in 1949, I was a very immature nineteen year-old "stud" who already knew a lot about everything. Ask me, if you have any doubts! The architecture of girls—and dates of that nature—interested me more than the architecture and dates of ancient buildings.

Pre-clinical studies would be at Pembroke College, third oldest college in Cambridge, founded by the Countess Pembroke in 1347. It is located in the center of a very old charming town, full of atmosphere.

Anatomy, physiology, pathology, biochemistry, organic chemistry, and pharmacology were my subjects of study, with an ultimate goal of a BA (Hons) degree. This I was to accomplish.

On that bright "first day" in October 1949, a taxi drove me from the Cambridge railway station to Pembroke College where a jovial Pembroke "porter" greeted me. He showed me to my room, explaining ground rules to me as we walked. (The only "rule" I can recall is that women had to be "Out" by 10:00 p.m.) Pembroke was a male college at that time, but today it is mixed and many of the rules have most likely changed.

We passed Christopher Wren's baroque chapel, and I'm ashamed to say that the only time I would visit Wren's Chapel was when I showed people around the College. Making our way to my room, I noted the library. It contained previous examination papers with important, valuable questions, the answers to which I would in due course commit to my photographic memory using "Windows 36."

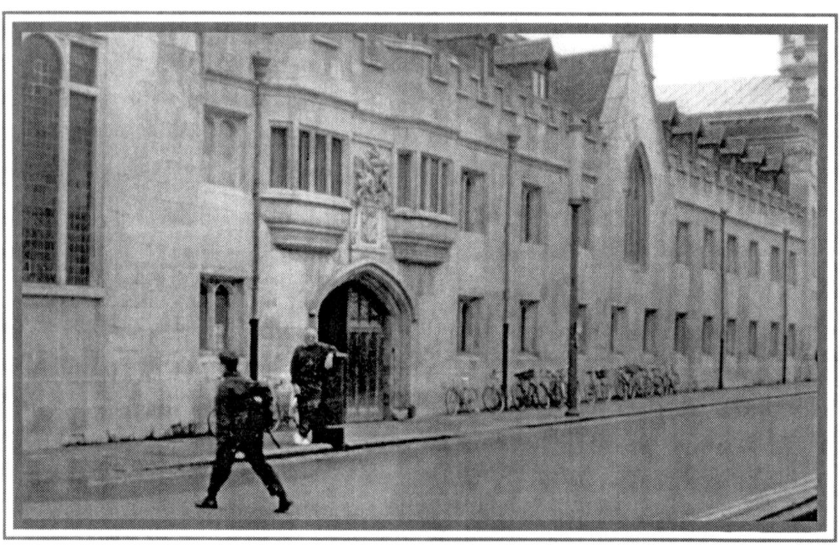

Pembroke College Main Entrance

The huge dining hall very much resembled that of Michaelhouse with its oil paintings of previous masters, deans and rectors. The portraits all held that familiar pompous, stuffy, superior expression. On first gathering in the dining hall, smiles on the faces of the good old colonial students from Australia, South Africa and other British countries visibly faded when they first set eyes on the solemn portraits.

A day or two after my arrival I strolled down to the Mill Pub located beside the River Cam, which meanders through the "backs" of various colleges. The pub is a short walk from Pembroke, and the River Cam would be the place to enjoy punting and picnicking with friends in the summer days ahead.

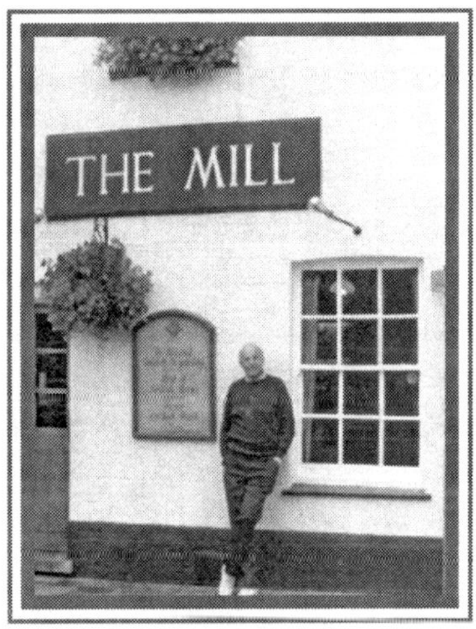

The Mill Pub

At Mill Pub, I had my first taste of English beer. Ah, yes, how quickly one becomes keen for that lukewarm bitter ale.

There are actually numerous pubs in Cambridge. A famous one was the "Eagle," which was frequented during the Second World War by pilots from nearby air stations. On the ceilings of the Eagle in black charcoal lettering, were the names of pilots and other armed forces soldiers who had enjoyed many a lukewarm English beer. Since many did not survive the war, they would never be privy to the honor given them.

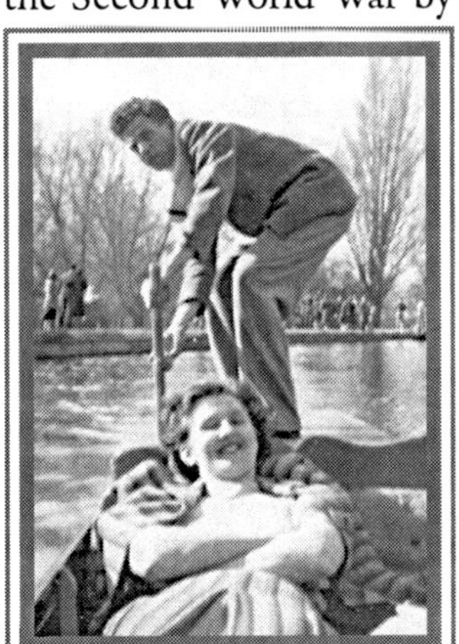
Punting on the River Cam

The town of Cambridge was, in some ways, separated from the colleges. In the Center, one could find some excellent curry restaurants. Curry is as popular in England as Mexican food is in the Southwest United States.

Students often congregated at Dorothy Café in the afternoons for so-called "tea dances." Dorothy Café was a somewhat sophisticated pick-up joint where students could enjoy high tea and pretend to be a Gene Kelly or Fred Astaire—much like the popular "Dancing with the Stars" of later years.

I immediately discovered that the bed in my room at Pembroke was much like sleeping on a slab of cement! Upon hearing of my wretched bed problem, my parents sent a six-foot, six-inch, non-collapsible bed—all the way from South Africa. I was still their pampered darling little Ian!

University life began in earnest. Students were soon absorbed in the daily routine of classes, studying, classes, and more studying.

Daniel Whylie was a fellow student who could easily have got me sent down (expelled). Whylie came from British aristocracy—or so he led us to believe—and was always immaculately dressed. He frequently wore a "trilby hat" (turned up at the sides) and spoke perfect King's English, or was it Queen's? Unlike the peculiar (cockney?) English spoken today. Real Pukka stuff!

The incident took place in a laboratory during a final exam. Alphabetically, Whyte and Whylie were seated side by side at a lab bench. Out of the corner of his mouth, Whylie asked me the answer to one of the questions. I pretended not to hear him. (Had I answered, and been seen by an invigilator, I could have quite easily been accused of cheating and sent down, thus ending my medical career.)

Bicycles were commonly used to get around the university campus, with baskets on the front to carry our books. It was quite convenient. Even our professor of pathology, "Daddy Dean," rode his bike to and from his lectures! He was ninety years old. (Probably what kept him young?)

Early on, I became involved in sports. While at Michaelhouse, I had been captain of our house athletic team. My best time for half-mile was 2 minutes and 7 seconds, but I felt I could improve on that with serious training and attain at least a half-blue. (One received a "blue" by representing Cambridge against Oxford, in any sport.)

Unfortunately, while I was training at Fenners one day, I sustained a classical Achilles tendon rupture! The trauma, however, went undiagnosed. It had me limping around for a year, putting a disappointing end to my sporting career.

All studies and no play makes Jack a dull boy. Shortly after arrival at Pembroke, I noted three pretty young women emerging with a young man from his room. An uneven number—3 to 1! I smoothed my hair, cleared my throat, and approached them with my most engaging smile.

We exchanged introductions, and the young man told me his name was John Reynolds. He introduced his beautiful sister, Laila, and her two girlfriends.

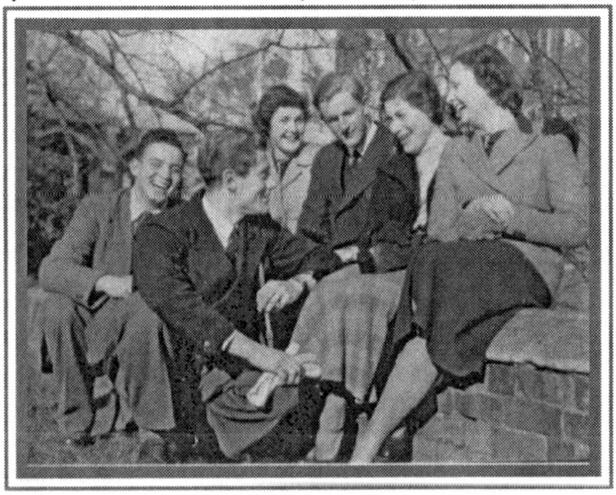

Ian, John, Tom, Laila and Friends at the "Bridge of Sighs"

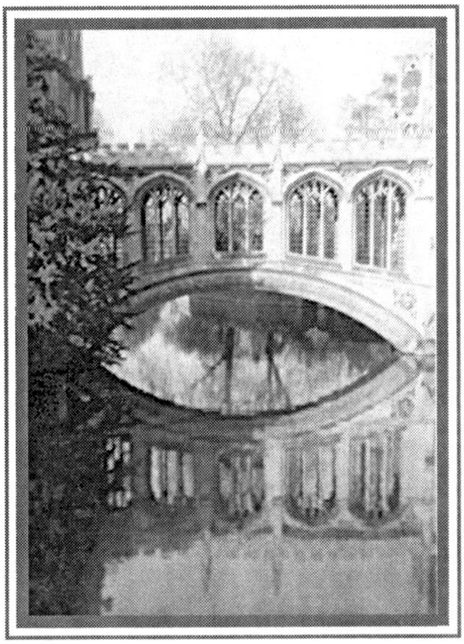

Bridge of Sighs

John was half-Russian and half-French. He had enlisted with the RAF (Royal Air Force) shortly before the end of the war, and received a RAF scholarship to Pembroke where he studied modern languages. He was to earn a "double-first" in French and Russian by the end of the first year. (Russian interpreters were in great demand to translate sensitive material.)

John and I became very good friends. He was a consummate Continental, with a sexy French

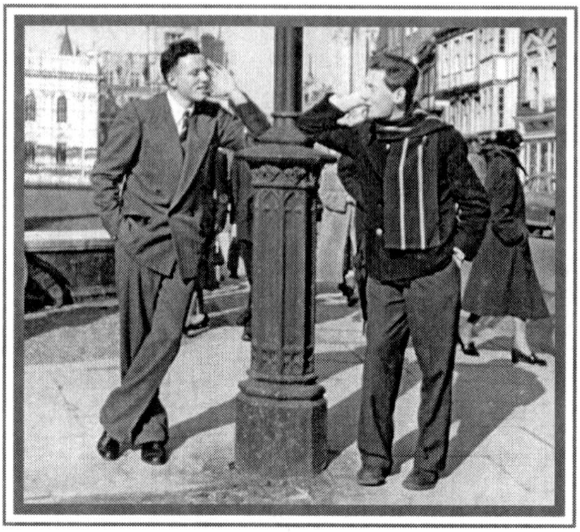

John Reynolds and Ian, Kings Parade

accent, and had the enviable knack of attracting good-looking women. (I was not too proud to accept some of his castaways.) Some of John's women friends came from the London stage, some from Dorothy Café, and various other places.

John and Laila had an interesting background. Born in Russia, their father was a Canadian playboy and their mother soon left him because of his philandering and infidelities. She had a tough time raising two small children without any financial support.

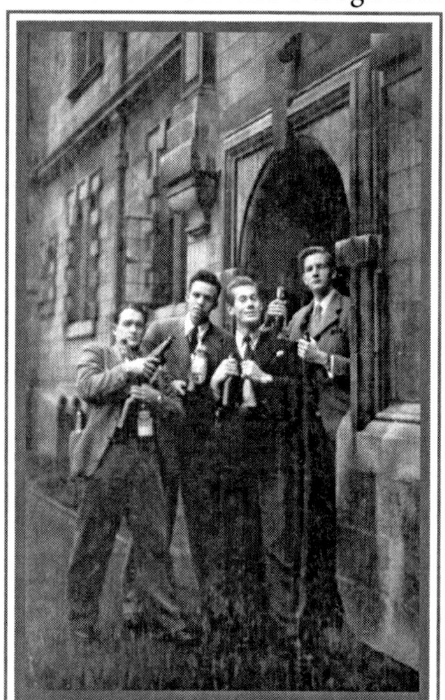

Pembroke Drinking Buddies

They were living in Europe, but moved to France at the outbreak of World War Two where they spent the duration under German occupation. John's mother soon fell in love with a French resistance fighter.

The Germans were encountering more and more resistance. They rounded up fifty Frenchmen, including the lover of John's mother, and shot them all. This was heart breaking to her. At the end of the war she moved with her children to England.

I was to meet both John's mother and granny in London—lovely people.

John and I once went down to London for a long weekend. John knew quite a few people in the Russian community and introduced me to a beautiful twenty-three year-old half Greek, half Russian, girl named Katrina. Her husband Reggie was an Oxford lawyer and a severe alcoholic. On occasion, Reggie would bring prostitutes back to their home.

John and Francesca (his girlfriend at the time), Katarina, Reggie, and I had dined at our favorite Indian curry restaurant, "Vera Swammy," on Regent Street, and we went on to Churchill's Nightclub. It was well after two a.m. when John and Francesca left us. Nobody was feeling much pain. Katrina, Reggie, and I went back to their cottage in Chelsea.

Reggie was plastered out of his mind and we managed to put him to bed. Shortly after I retired, there was a knock on my guest bedroom door, and Katrina jumped into bed with me. This was the first time I had ever slept with a married woman, never mind one having a husband in the room next door! We could hear his noisy snoring, so I was reasonably sure there would be little chance of coitus interrupt-us!

Months later, John told me Katrina was a nymphomaniac. Her problem was failure to ever experience orgasm. She went from man to man looking for Mr. Wonderful. Needless to say, I did not qualify.

A year later, Reggie was involved in a fatal car accident while drunk, having slammed into a tree.

An influx of students from all over converged on Cambridge during the summer months, anxious to learn English. Amongst these, certain beautiful Swedish women caught my eye and I came up with a brilliant idea to teach English—or Zulu, if one preferred!—to these incoming students. (No need for them to know I could not read.)

Soon my notice went up on the bulletin boards: "Expert English lessons taught in the Cromwell Study—free!" (The Cromwell Study was my room.)

In 1615, Oliver Cromwell entered Sydney Sussex College, Cambridge at the age of seventeen. He did not obtain a Cambridge degree as he was more interested in athletics than studies. There was considerable speculation as to whether or not my bedroom had been his. (The mattress surely felt like it. But may we leave it at that?)

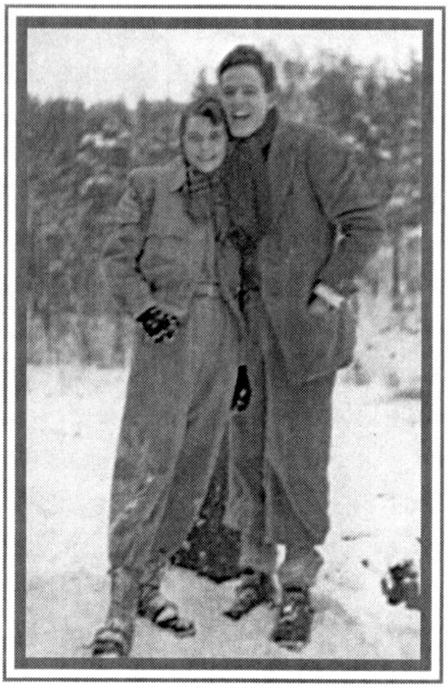
Gunilla and Ian

Soon I had a small flock of students, all eager to learn English within the prestigious walls of my (and Cromwell's?) bedroom. Gunilla was one such student—a tall, slender brunette from Gothenburg, Sweden.

Lovely Gunilla invited me to her home for Christmas to meet her parents, and to continue her English lessons. During this time, we attended a student gathering at the University of Lund in Malmo to celebrate "Santa Lucia." The students attending were all dressed in white, including white caps, and went to visit their professors. An interesting event.

The Swedish smorgasbord was a delight! During the war, Sweden had remained neutral and as a result had an abundance of food. (On the other hand, Cambridge still had various rationed items—sugar, eggs, butter, and sweets. This, mind you, was 1950—five years after the war ended!)

By the conclusion of Christmas holiday, Gunilla spoke magnificent English—with a South African accent. I had learned a smattering of rudimentary Swedish, including many Swedish toasts. Toasts were made prior to gulping down shots of Schnapps. "Min skal, din skal, alla vakra flickor skal." Translated, "My toast, your toast, a toast to all the beautiful women." The Schnapps burned all the way down to the tips of one's toes.

What a lovely Christmas, which ended all too soon.

Cambridge students occupied rooms within the college for the first year only. After that, we were obliged to find our own "digs" somewhere outside the college, preferably not too far from where the lectures were held. As a result, I changed my digs after year one.

I rented a room in the home of newlyweds Lillian and Bruce Whitby-Stevens on the outskirts of Cambridge. Lillian was a comely redhead with bright blue eyes. Bruce resembled a naughty, rosy-cheeked little English schoolboy. They had been married barely six months.

On the second floor, my bedroom was adjacent to theirs. The sounds of their nightly antics (frequent agonizing screams and banging against the headboard) were certainly a diversion from Grey's Anatomy! I refrained from calling the local police, although it had actually crossed my mind.

England's King George VI died on February 6, 1952. Since I was not a dyed-in-the-wool Englander, the event held little interest to me. Busily going about my business that solemn English day, I was whistling to myself. Lillian heard me and was outraged. She gave me merry hell for whistling.

I say, the Brits certainly take these things seriously.

John Reynolds introduced me to an extremely pretty young woman, a dancer on the London stage whose stage name was "Gay Pearl."

Gay Pearl visited me at Pembroke one day, and we were soon dancing naked and cheek to cheek to "Bewitched, Bothered and Bewildered," popularly sung by Doris Day.

I noticed that Gay had a most fantastic figure. "I'm wild again, beguiled again, a simpering, whimpering child again. Bewitched, bothered, and bewildered am I. Couldn't sleep, and wouldn't sleep, when love came and told me . . ." Suddenly, I remembered that I had an exam appointment in precisely three minutes, almost forgotten by me in my absorption of the moment! I reluctantly left Gay in my room and dashed off to the 3:00 on-the-nose anatomy exam.

There were two examiners, the first being a Dr. Jack Harris who handed me a bone and asked, "What is this?"

"Sir, this is an old fibula." (I use the word "old" quite frequently in my ordinary conversation as a term of endearment, such as "old friend.") My answer produced a laugh from the examiners, and then Dr. Harris continued.

"What is inserted here?"

"Flexor Hallucis Longus."

"Here?

"Peroneus brevis."

"And here?"

"Flexor digitorum longus."

The examiner went over the entire fibula. It was a piece of cake—all neatly laid out in my photographic mind from page 415 of Grey's Anatomy!

Next, Dr. Harris produced a skull and pointed to the roof of the orbit where the eyeball sits.

"What is this?"

"The roof of the orbit is formed almost entirely by the orbital plate of the frontal bone (page 262)."

The viva (oral questioning) went on for about half an hour, and I managed to answer all of their questions.

The exam completed, I raced back to my room fully expecting to find Gay gone. But she was not. Off came our clothes, and we picked up where we left off.

"She may laugh, but I love it, although the laugh's on me..."

The first year at Cambridge had passed, and I returned to South Africa for the long vacation. Apartheid government was in full swing and crime was escalating.

On a late afternoon, I walked from nearby Howard College toward Manning Road, taking a shortcut on a dirt path surrounded by heavy bush. I had just gone off the path to take a leak behind a large tree when I heard terrible screaming coming from the direction of the path. Standing motionless, I peered cautiously out from behind the tree to observe what appeared to be a robbery.

It was payday, and two Africans had hidden in the bush, presumably waiting to rob someone. The unlucky someone was an African returning home from work. With a quick lethal blow from a machete, the poor fellow was almost decapitated.

The robbers went through the victim's pockets, and quickly removed his running shoes. Then they disappeared back into the bush. The poor bugger lay in a pool of blood on the dirt path. His head was at a grotesque angle and there was absolutely no doubt he was dead.

Frozen with fear, I was convinced that had the killers seen me (the only witness), I would also become history. Finally, I dashed home and phoned the police, telling them what I had seen and where the body was.

"Wragtig man, is die kerel dood?" ("No kidding, is the fellow dead?")

The police officer seemed disinterested, and I could detect aggravation in his voice. "Ag man! Nog n Blerrie Kaffir." ("Just another bloody Kaffir.")

Yes, South Africa was changing, and life was cheap.

My maternal grandmother's maiden name was Grant, and she was born in Fraserburgh, Scotland. I am not certain when or where she met my grandfather, a baker, but they married. My mother was soon born to them in Aberdeen, Scotland. In 1907, the family immigrated to South Africa. Many people were leaving Europe at the turn of the century because of grim conditions—economic hardship, famine, and God alone knows what else!

After grandfather died many, many years later, Granny came to live with my parents in Durban. She took over Lizzie's bedroom.

Granny loved to smoke in bed. (She claimed not to inhale the cigarettes.) A frail little creature, granny suffered from severe bronchitis and emphysema, and weighed barely ninety pounds.

Since the day she got off the ship in 1907, granny's Scottish accent had not changed one bit!

I decided to show off some colored slides to my parents and granny one evening—pictures of Cambridge, London, and Paris (where I had spent my first Christmas). In the slide presentation one of my Swedish English students, Inge, suddenly flashed onto the large screen. She was stark naked, wearing only my Pembroke scarf which I had casually draped around her pretty shoulders.

A bit embarrassed, I hurried on to the next slide, but granny had seen it and said, "I can see the wee bairn was having a good time." She then poured herself a not too "wee drap" of old Paarl K.W.V. brandy and lit up a Springbok cigarette.

Granny died at age eighty-nine of colonic cancer. My father, who was President of SAVES (South African Voluntary Euthanasia Society), made sure she did not suffer.

Mother was a free spirit, but seemed concerned about my risqué relationships. The slide show had roused her suspicions. She arranged for me to visit the venereal disease clinic at the black hospital, King Edward. There I saw the ravages of untreated syphilis—general paralysis of the insane, with every possible complication. Pretty gross stuff. Still, it was not enough to slow me down for too long!

The Christmas break to Paris in 1949—noted during my slide show—was taken alone. I decided to attend the Josephine Baker (1906-1975) performance at the Folies Bergere. (My father had seen Ms. Baker perform at the Follies some 25 years earlier, when she was age nineteen.)

Josephine Baker had an intriguing career for fifty years. I was intrigued that evening as I watched her descend the stairs in an enormous white flowing gown and her elaborate trademark headdress. The completely naked dancers in her show were gorgeous. I had never seen anything like this in my life—standing room only, to the very back of the theater.

Josephine Frida McDonald was born on June 3, 1906 of mixed ethnic parents. Her career began as a small girl dancing in the streets of Paris. In 1925, a Paris review acclaimed her an overnight success after her previous evening's erotic appearance wearing only high heels and a skirt made of bananas. It was the talk of the town.

The Folies Bergere became stomping grounds for Ms. Baker over the ensuing years. Her pet cheetah, named Chiquita, sometimes accompanied Josephine, always wearing a diamond collar. On occasion, Chiquita escaped into the orchestra pit, creating havoc with the musicians!

Josephine was involved in the French Underground Resistance movement during the Second World War, but she was so popular that the Nazis, who occupied Paris at that time, left her alone!

In the 1950's, Josephine was involved in the Civil Rights Movement. She adopted twelve multi-ethnic orphans whom she called her "rainbow tribe." She was quoted as saying, "We can all make our dreams come true, but first we have to decide to awaken from them."

Josephine Baker—a fascinating woman, and a spectacular singer and performer.

After leaving the Follies, I strolled back to my hotel room on Rue de Vaugirard in the Latin Quarter. Two young French girls approached me. Each took an arm and led me (not protesting) to a nearby hotel. It was there where I first laid eyes on a French bidet. The girls had me straddling the bidet, where they proceeded to carefully wash my privates! Though somewhat taken aback by all of this, I was young, curious, and possessed of many healthy "whoremoans!"

A very quick 20 francs later, I left the hotel room. Such open promiscuity was unheard of in South Africa, where even Playboy Magazine was outlawed!

In Paris, I met a fellow medical student. Nihal Ranasinghe was from Ceylon and a student at Clare College, Cambridge. We spent time together in Paris and became good friends.

A tiny fellow, Nihal told me he could squeeze himself through the bars of his college bedroom window. Quite an interesting revelation. By approximating his shoulders, he was able to wiggle through the window—a great asset because we had to be in our rooms by 10:00 p.m. or the "proctor" (campus police, Cambridge style) would be after us.

Fifty years later (in 2005), I located Nihal through the internet and telephoned him. He was living in Kandy, a town in the middle of Ceylon now called Sri Lanka. His father and grandfather were medical men who had also attended Clare College, Cambridge, and his son was about to graduate as a medical doctor, as well. Unfortunately, Nihal was suffering with Parkinson's disease.

We had a pleasant visit over the telephone that day. Nihal had no trouble remembering me, the wild South African he had met in Paris fifty years earlier.

There were a few relatively short vacations during the school year. The Dominion Trust Foundation organized by one Lady Cynthia Campbell of Argyleshire, a kindly Scottish dowager duchess, placed Dominion students in various lovely homes all over England and Scotland during our short breaks. Several interviews were arranged to screen Colonials in order to ensure we were fit to not embarrass the people whose homes we would visit. (I recall that black students were conspicuous by their absence from these parties.)

One of my visits was to the west coast of Scotland. The Glen, Ardgour, Argylshire, home of Mrs. Beatrice Stapleton. This magnificent estate was located very near Scotland's highest mountain, Ben Nevis.

Mrs. Stapleton was an extremely wealthy woman. Her hunting, shooting and fishing lodge would, many years later, be host to visitors such as Lady Diana and Prince Charles.

Our dinners were served by a young German housekeeper at an enormous refectory table, easily seating 20 people! Most often there was

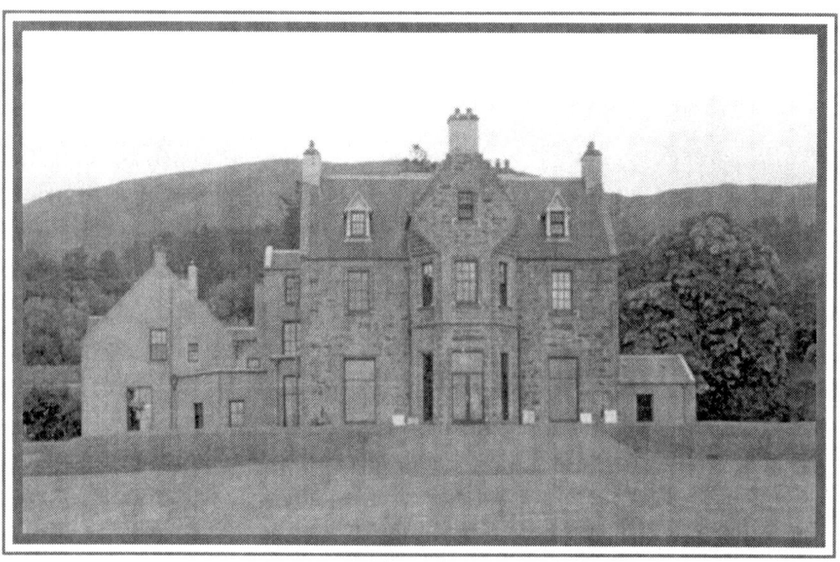

Conaglen

just the two of us—Beatrice at the one end, young Ian at the other, and a great expanse of long table in-between. The table was laden with delectables, and I recall especially the enormous delicious strawberries.

Beatrice's estate was the site of excellent salmon fishing. The game warden, Bruce, had a peculiar method of catching salmon. He dropped a line with a barbed hook into the clear water right next to the salmon, and gave the line a jerk. This may have been illegal, but I suppose anything goes if the property is private. The salmon was scrumptious.

Lady Biddiford's home in Buckinghamshire was another of these short vacations.

Alighting from the bus outside of the appointed address, I noticed a small house quite near the roadside. Approaching, I wondered with bewilderment if this might be where I would be staying. It was, in fact, only the gatehouse! (The main home was about two hundred yards further up a winding road.)

It was past eleven a.m. when I arrived. Lady Riddiford was a most gracious hostess, and offered me a "Pimms Number 1." It did not stop at one!

Also staying with Lady Riddiford at the time was a Swiss exchange student, a young girl who spoke perfect English. We became friends, and she would later visit me at Cambridge.

We punted on the Cam River with others and took a picnic to a lovely sleepy little village, Grantchester. Grantchester was home of the famous English post, Rupert Brooke. His poem, "The Old Vicarage, Grantchester," concludes with these famous words: "Here stands the church clock at 10 to 3. And is there still honey for tea?" Believe it or not, the church clock's hands at Grantchester still stand at 10 to 3.

At the beginning of World War One, Rupert Brooke wrote a sad poem called, "The Soldier." The poem's final lines ring a rather sad note. "If I should die, think only this of me, that there's some corner of a foreign field forever England. Cheer up, chaps, there are three lovely pubs just around the corner!"

It was on one of our longer summer holidays that Mike, a Pembroke cricket blue, and I went to Europe, visiting France and Italy.

In Rome, the highlight of our visit was to 64 Via Veneto, a magnificent bordello (house of prostitution).

Our taxi pulled up to the front entrance, and we walked up a marble staircase to the first floor. We were greeted by an attractive woman in her forties who ushered us to a large waiting room. The room held life-sized replicas of Venus de Milo and Michelangelo's David, and comfortable seats surrounded a fountain in the middle of the room.

Madam spoke perfect English, and after a short introduction she ushered in several beautiful young women. Each was dressed scantily in see-through negligees. There were blondes, brunettes, and redheads. Some were tall, some petite, some thin, some not so thin. Certainly, it was a selection to please the most capricious of clients.

Mike chose a large blonde German woman and they immediately disappeared into inner sanctum. On the other hand, I was inhibited as usual by my "condition," and reluctant to participate. I remained seated. Madam understood and offered me porno magazines to arouse my libido—but no luck.

Three police officers suddenly entered the house—to make an arrest, I was certain. This was, after all, a house of prostitution! The thought of spending a night in jail in Rome was not appealing. But the police wanted only to check our passports!

I began to wonder what was keeping Mike so long when he suddenly walked into the room. "What in God's name have you been doing?" I asked!

"Let's get out of here quick, and I'll tell you," he said.

His "approach" to the young German prostitute was apparently offensive, and she did not like the way Mike was going about things. After much aerobic exercise, Madam appeared in the room. She returned his money, and then kicked him out.

The ferry from Sorrento took us to the magical island of Capri. Approaching the island, one has the impression of a large rock jutting from the ocean waters.

Mike and I climbed from the harbor to the top with our rucksacks. It was quite a challenge. We arrived at the old landmark hotel, the Grand Hotel Quisiana, in the picturesque town Square. Tables with checkered tablecloths and brightly colored umbrellas were scattered on the sidewalk. We sat down and ordered a cappuccino.

Sitting at the table next to us was a most attractive blond, and introductions soon followed. Her name was Stephanie. She was an American, visiting Capri to get away from New York where she had just been through a nasty divorce. Her son was off visiting his father. Stephanie must have been at least ten years older than us.

Stephanie joined us at our table, and Mike ordered a couple of bottles of Torciano Brunella Di Montalcino (the worldwide darling of the wine connoisseur). For the first time our surly waiter actually smiled!

Stephanie asked if we would care to stay with her at her villa. It was an offer we could not refuse. The villa was located on a high hillside overlooking the blue Mediterranean, and we spent the entire week there. Stephanie was a warm and lovely lady, and we had a memorable time.

The Blue Grotto is a place everyone who visits Capri must see. It is the emblem of the island. Reportedly, Roman emperors who once had villas on Capri used the Blue Grotto as a private bath.

The Grotto can be reached only by small rowboats through a partially submerged opening into the sea. A separate entrance is completely submerged by the water. Sunlight reflects off the limestone bottom of the Grotto (cave), illuminating the water from below and giving it an intense color of blue. It is truly a spectacular sight which I am sure "turned on" the old emperors!

Near Stephanie's villa was the home of Gracie Field, well-known English actress whose lovely singing voice brought her from rags to riches. On Capri, Gracie could find brief refuge from the public eye. She offered us the use of her private swimming area, the culmination of our week on the lovely island of Capri.

It was soon time to leave. As the ferryboat drew away from the small harbor of Marina Grande, Mike and I waved a sad farewell to Stephanie who stood on the jetty. As she became smaller and smaller and then was gone from sight, the words of an old lyric played music in my head:

"T'was on the Isle of Capri that I found her, beneath the shade of an old walnut tree. Oh, I can still see the flowers around her, where we met on the Isle of Capri."

Cambridge finals were fast approaching, and we students spent many long hours in our rooms with intense studying. While I still could not read a complete sentence without stumbling, my blackboard visual aid allowed access to my photographic memory.

Most of my information came from small shortened textbooks (aids to every subject). I summarized this material, and then made shorter versions to photograph (in my Windows 36). While I attended the lectures, they were not of much help to me.

The Cambridge tutorial system was excellent, and the teachers were some of the finest. It was a unique tutorial system, and involved two or three students getting together with a teacher for one hour, several times a week. One could learn a great deal this way.

Examinations came and went. To my immense pleasure and relief, I received my BA Hons (cantab) degree.

I had applied to St. Thomas' Hospital in London for the next (clinical) portion of my medical training (still a medical student, but without patient contact). "Tommy's" had the reputation of being the best-dressed hospital in London. I was hardly an impressive "clothes horse" and I'm afraid Tommy's fashion-mindedness never rubbed off on me.

The old boy network was a great help with my interview at St. Thomas. Dad knew the chief anesthesiologist, Dr. Sam Lawrence. Just before the interview, Sam visited me in the waiting room and gave me a briefing.

"How many languages do you speak?"

"Four languages—English, Afrikaans, Zulu, and Russian."

"That's just what the doctors like to hear," Sam said. (Heaven only knows why.) Nonetheless, in my interview I spoke some fancy Zulu—and added several impressive clicking sounds, for effect.

I was in! St. Thomas accepted me for three years of clinical training (1952-1955).

Before concluding my memoirs of Cambridge University, I would like to recount the interesting life story of my friend, John Reynolds.

John's sister, Laila, moved to Paris to work as an executive secretary at the exclusive George V Hotel. There she met Rudolf (Rudy) Lieberman, son of the founder of Symantic Welding, a cold welding process company. Upon the death of his father, Rudy became a multimillionaire with franchises all over the globe.

Laila and Rudy married and lived in their Fifth Avenue penthouse in New York. Other residences were in Monaco, Switzerland, and their 100 ft. yacht in the Greek island of Corfu.

I met Rudy and Laila briefly at the Ritz-Carlton Hotel in Montreal in 1957. Rudy was a bald, rotund little man, somewhat lacking in personality, I thought. Yet, they did seem to be in love. Laila, the penniless young woman who, with her mother and brother John, went from France to England after the war, was now a very wealthy woman. It was certainly a rags-to-riches story.

In 1958, Laila and Rudy had a son and named him Alan. Shortly after, Laila drove her Ferrari to a New York airport to meet her mother who was coming in from London for Alan's christening. She was quite suddenly the victim of a dreadful car accident, and died five days later from massive head injuries.

Reportedly, Laila had previously taken out a life insurance policy for $75,000, making her mother the beneficiary. In 1958, this was a lot of money. Rudy felt the money should be his but Laila's brother, John, said "No way." A tremendous falling out followed, and their mother was ultimately awarded the $75,000.

John was entrusted with the money by his mother, and he handled it wisely. Over the course of the next twenty years, they became multi-millionaires with many apartment buildings in Manhattan and several beautiful homes in Southampton.

Laila's son, Alan, grew up, married, and had four children. The family lived in a town close to the Swiss/French border. When Alan was thirty-five, his name appeared in a Swiss magazine as one of nine of the wealthiest men in Switzerland! This was, perhaps, the incident that later led trouble to his door.

On the fateful day, Alan's wife and four children were away for a few days. Alan was home alone when two men on a motorcycle arrived and forced their way inside the house. A terrifying skirmish followed. Alan was no match for the men and suffered multiple wounds from a stiletto knife. They tied him up, gagged him, threw him to the back floor of his BMW, and covered him with a sheet.

Off they drove. Alan recalls crossing the Swiss/French border and going through Customs. He begged the kidnappers to loosen his hands, as his badly cut hand was giving him intense pain. The sheet was causing breathing difficulty. Finally relenting, the kidnappers loosened the ties and removed the sheet.

Darkness set in, and Alan managed to untie his wrists and ankles. He soon had the window partially cracked open. When the car paused at a stop light, Alan threw himself out the open window but his foot became stuck. The car gained speed. Alan wiggled loose, fell out the window, and was thrown into a ditch.

Covered in blood, he walked to a nearby farmhouse where he saw lights coming from within. He knocked and a farmer opened the door, but slammed it shut after one look at Alan's bloody face.

Alan found refuge in the farmer's barn and hid behind a bale of hay. Later that night, he heard the voices of the kidnappers who had returned to search for him. They did not find him, and by morning all was quiet. He made his way to town to report the incident to the police.

Inquires were made by the police and it was discovered that the kidnappers had recently rented a small farmhouse in the vicinity. The place was raided and police found a ransom note for ten million francs in exchange for Alan's life!

The rogues were soon captured and sentenced to ten years in a French prison. Quite a story!

St. Thomas' Hospital, London, 1952. The three years of medical school at St. Thomas' Hospital were vitally important because they laid the foundation for excellent medical training in medicine, surgery, gynecology, obstetrics, and pediatrics. Since I could still not read, I had to put in countless hours with my brain's Windows 36.

I arrived in London a somewhat more mature man than when I had arrived in Cambridge a few years earlier. The city was cold, and often damp and rainy. A tremendous fog sometimes arose in the winter so badly that one could barely see a few feet ahead.

My first task was to locate living accommodations. In the London Times' advertisement section, I found an ad for a Mews cottage at 5 pounds a week, heating and electricity extra.

At 35, Huntsworth Mews, off Ivor Place, Glouchester Street, the address was very near Baker Street's underground station and would be an easy ride to St. Thomas' Hospital. The quaint, two-story building was converted from old stables and the Mews had a cobblestone street. I noted a cheery blue window box protruding from the upstairs window. Inside, two tiny bedrooms and a small kitchen comprised the apartment.

Peter, my old "Elephant 8" buddy who was studying engineering in London, would be sharing the apartment with me and paying half of the rent. Because of the very cold winter weather, the gas heater gobbled up shillings at a great rate.

Living below us was the landlady, Mrs. Myra Burnside, and her ancient maid, Dolly. We could often hear heated arguments coming from downstairs, particularly when Dolly refused to take her weekly bath.

Mrs. Burnside had a large African gray parrot by the name of Toby. Toby talked with an Oxford accent and often said, "You show me yours, old boy, and I will show you mine." Toby could also recite a series of expletives much too obscene to repeat here!

And so, Peter and I soon settled into our tiny apartment, which would be our home for the coming three years.

London is a lovely old city, despite the weather. St. Thomas' Hospital was, in 1215, already described as ancient! You do the counting. It is located on the Thames' south embankment opposite the Houses of Parliament and Big Ben, with London Bridge located nearby. During the Second World War, the hospital had suffered extensive damage, but repairs were made by the time I arrived in October of 1952.

Nearby, the Florence Nightingale School of Nursing and Midwifery at St. Thomas'—established in 1860—is regarded as a center of excellence in its field. The many attractive nurses attending the school wore white uniforms and pert white caps, and this certainly added interest to the entire learning experience.

During the course of my studies at Tommy's, I came down with a nasty case of Infectious Mononucleosis, the kissing disease, and I was briefly hospitalized. My consultant, Sir Forrest-Hill, felt that because my name is spelled with a "y", I must be related to a famous Surrey golfer! When I told him I thought not, he immediately lost interest in my case!

On another occasion, I developed mumps and the bug traveled to my testicles causing high fever, deliriums, and hallucinations. My consultant, Dr. Robert McGinty, thought I was worried about future offspring. With extremely painful and enormously swollen testicles, offspring was the last thing on my mind!

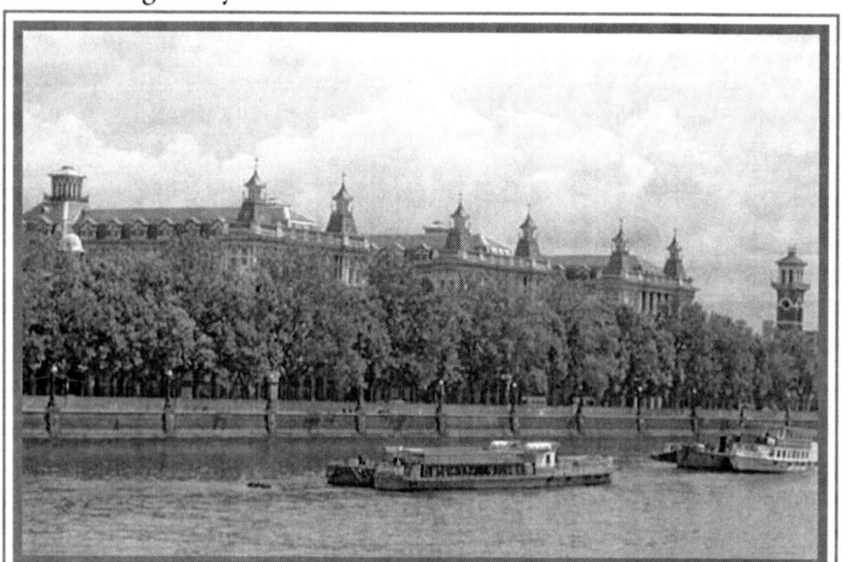

St. Thomas's Hospital

The busy days soon became routine, with intense devotion to studies. Consultants at Tommy's taught students to listen carefully to the patient because, in doing so, the patient will often give the doctor the diagnosis. Observation of the patient, careful history taking, and a meticulous physical examination are all followed by the ordering of appropriate tests.

Alas! With the advances in medicine today, doctors too quickly go for the envelope with the x-rays!

I received hands-on experience at Tommys' by observing how things should be done and gaining the tools that would carry me through the next thirty-five years of medical practice.

The hospital library contained old examination papers with very relevant important questions, and I often visited. I would print my answers in indelible ink into my memory.

I really came into my own here, and my dyslexia was much less bothersome than in previous years. Strange though it may seem, I never ever thought of myself in any way as disabled.

It was during this timeframe that I visited a spinal injury center at Stoke Manderville, where Dr. Samuel Guttman was a foremost authority in the treatment of paraplegics and quadriplegics. Later knighted because of his brilliant work, he became Sir Samuel Guttman.

It was amazing to witness patients rehabilitated at the center, and to watch paraplegics taught how to walk using spinal accessory muscles. Most of the serious spinal injuries came from automobile accidents.

A South African patient at the center—who had dived into an empty swimming pool—was a quadriplegic. I had a long talk with him, wishing him well, but knowing that his future would be an uphill battle. These are catastrophic injuries.

While lunching in the center's cafeteria, I felt a tap on my shoulder. It was Mike, the man with the big weapon whom I had fled from in the Turkish bath in London! I felt cornered into having lunch with him, and he asked me if I would like to spend the night with him! His kind invitation was politely declined as I once again bid him adieu, and moved quickly in the direction of the door!

London House is located in Russell Square, a residence where many overseas and postgraduate students lived. Some wild parties took place here. It was at one of these parties in October of 1952 that I met an engineering student, Bertie Krantz, who was to become a life-long friend.

Bertie was born in Harbor Island in the Bahamas. Although an extraordinary man with many distinctive achievements in his life, he was also the ultimate ladies' man. In years to come, Bertie was known to have mistresses in Monte Carlo, London (a young Finnish woman who was also the mistress of a lord), and in Vienna. He also had a twenty year affair with his neighbor's beautiful wife, Karen.

Bertie must have been a chip off the old block. His father died in Switzerland at age sixty-two in the arms of a nineteen year-old. Bertie flew to Switzerland to make funeral arrangements, and to comfort the nineteen year old!

It was at this same party I met Lisa Wilson. Lisa was a blond knockout nurse from St. Mary's Hospital in London. She would later become my first wife. Lisa was dating Fred Blake at the time, one of my old oversexed Michaelhouse buddies. When he returned to South Africa several weeks later, Lisa and I began to date in a relatively monogamous fashion.

During obstetric training in Guilford, a pretty little village in Surrey, Lisa missed a period. I had been through this before, so I immediately performed a "frog test." A female frog is injected with a woman's urine. If the test is positive (pregnant), the frog will ovulate. I wanted to witness results for myself, and what I saw was the huge frog floating in a sea of eggs! The frog looked at me with critical eyes, as if to say, "Boy, are you are in deep shit now."

Lisa was pregnant. I was about one year from my final exams—and now had a pregnant girlfriend! Marriage did not seem an option, so I arranged for an abortion for Lisa in London with an ethical abortionist, if there is such an individual.

But when the time came, I could not let Lisa go through with it. I really loved her

We told her parents, Stuart and Vera. Lisa was their only child and her father turned ashen at the news. My own father was furious. He would finance us, he announced, until the baby was born and until I qualified. From then on we were on our own, and he meant it.

My mother was a depressed, anxious woman under normal circumstances. The marriage fiasco precipitated what was tantamount to a nervous breakdown. I managed to get a psychologist to see her for a couple of sessions before the wedding, and had a session myself!

Perhaps this was an example of the old saying, "Youth is wasted on the young." But we make our mistakes and move on.

The wedding took place on August 7, 1954 in a little chapel just outside of Amersham in Buckinghamshire. It was a lovely sunny day, not your typical English weather.

The church service was brief, and invited guests were only family and close friends. Colin Visser (my gay friend from South Africa) was my best man, and mother flew over from South Africa. Dad had no intention of attending!

After the service, Lisa and I drove off for a brief honeymoon at Henley, a small picturesque town where Oxford and Cambridge have their annual boat races. I will never forget the parting words to me from Lisa's mother as we drove off in our rented Mini Minor—"I hope you have better luck with Lisa than we did!" In retrospect, that should have told me something.

Lisa was only seven years old when she was evacuated to Canada during the war, as were many English children. The bombing of London had become grim and the Wilsons felt this was a wise choice. These were difficult times for children, and her Canadian adoptive parents had many problems with her acting out.

We returned from our honeymoon. Peter moved out of our Mews and Lisa moved in. Peter had never liked Lisa, for reasons I only found out much later on. Apparently she had made several passes at him!

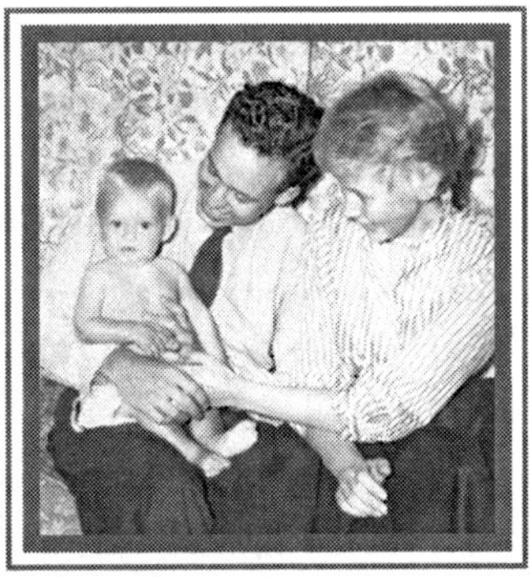

Doting Parents

And so, our married life began under very depressing circumstances. Our son, Wilson, was born on February 15, 1955 in Westminster Hospital. He was somewhat yellow at birth and while he did not look like either of us, I was reasonably sure I was the father. Never in a million years did either Lisa or I foresee that Wilson would develop paranoid schizophrenia in his later teenage years. An absolute heartbreak for any parent.

The Cambridge final medical exams came in June 1955, and I FAILED. It was a bitter blow. The fact that fifty-five percent of my class failed as well was of little comfort to me.

The main reason I failed was because of one question—"Discuss the surgery of the thymus gland." It was a question that had never ever come up before in any Cambridge final.

In humans, the thymus is a soft flattened pinkish-grey organ located in the upper chest under the breastbone. It grows throughout childhood up to the age of puberty, and then gradually decreases in size and blends with the surrounding tissue.

This "question" should never have been in a medical final qualifying exam. Possibly in a higher surgical degree?

In the written surgery paper there were four questions, no choices, and all had to be answered in essay form. If one did poorly in just one of the questions, one had to do exceptionally well in the rest of the exam in order to pass. Well, I thought that maybe I had!

I went to see Sir Lionel Whitby, Chancellor of Cambridge University and co-author of the English bible of hematology entitled "Whitby and Briton."

At my request, Sir Lionel kindly looked into the matter and ultimately found that one of the two examiners had failed me. There were only two examiners, and to this day I am puzzled as to why, if those two could not decide, a third was not introduced!

Can you imagine this scenario? A dyslexic South African student who is unable to read debates convincingly with Sir Lionel, the Chancellor of Cambridge University. Dyslexia in no way affected my ability to speak!

The next opportunity to take this exam would be in December, six months later. For those six months, I applied myself diligently to my studies.

Lisa's figure returned to normal after Wilson was born, and Steve Hart, President of Tommys' camera club, approached her to see if she would consider doing some modeling. We decided the idea was good, especially as the club would pay five pounds a shoot.

There were only two requirements: Nude models must 1) remove all pubic hair; and 2) sign a release acknowledging that the photos taken by Steve in his home would remain his property. What he did with them was at his sole discretion.

Steve was a very wealthy (family money) roly-poly teddy bear type, with a heart of gold. The club met every second Thursday, and the sessions lasted the better part of two hours.

At twenty-two, Lisa was gorgeous and the shoots were going well. After she had modeled for the club a number of times, Steve invited her to accompany them on a long weekend in the Scilly Islands for a shoot—all expenses paid.

Lisa called me from her luxurious hotel, the "Hell Bay Inn" in the Scilly Isles, excited about the whole thing. She described the hotel, the secluded private sandy beach situated right on the seafront, and her suite which was beautifully furnished with sculptures and paintings by local artists.

When the shoots were completed, Lisa returned home a bit richer.

Steve invited us to his home for lunch shortly after the shoot. His home was located in the most affluent part of Chelsea, beautifully appointed, with an elegant living room and a dining room with a large old refectory table. His bedroom was warm and inviting with original period furniture, mirrors on several walls and ceiling—all looking like the work of an interior decorator. (Unbeknownst to me, Lisa had seen herself in those mirrors in her birthday suit.)

After a delicious lunch, Steve presented Lisa with a leather bound portfolio of photographs taken in the Scilly Isles, half black and white and half in color, printed from slides. Lisa looked stunning, the photographs superb. Most of the colored photos were shot on the beach with its pure white sand and the blue Atlantic in the background.

One photo was of the group's farewell picnic on the beach. It showed four camera club bachelors in swimsuits, arms around stark-naked Lisa, toasting Cardinal Puff in the hopes of becoming a "cardinal!" This is a sophisticated form of binge drinking, quite prevalent at the time. The slightest deviation from the script or actions will require the candidate to stop, down his or her beer, buy the next round, and start again.

"Here's to the health of Cardinal Puff, swallow one gulp of beer, wipe mustache with one finger on each side, once. Here's to the health of Cardinal Puff for the second time, swallow two gulps of beer, wipe mustache with two fingers on each side twice. Here's to the health of Cardinal Puff for the third and last time, swallow the rest of the beer, wipe mustache with three fingers on each side, thrice. Put down the beer mug upside down on the table, belch loudly, and say, "I am a Cardinal."

All cardinals are eligible to become members of the Ancient Order of Froth Blowers, a very old "venereal" society!

The camera club group looked so young and carefree facing Steve's camera, with happy tipsy-smiles. Steve was kind and protective of Lisa. Much older than the rest of us, he was considered an "institute" at Thomas'—the perpetual student.

Lisa was paid fifty pounds for the three-day shoot, which was a fortune in those days. She and I bought Steve a present as a thank-you—a ceramic creation of a large pink pig, beautifully done. In retrospect, because Steve was grossly overweight, the gift was not the kindest or well thought out selection!

Lisa continued to model for the club until we left for Canada.

In December, I wrote my Cambridge final, and this time passed with flying colors. Sir John Robertson (Prime Minister Harold Macmillan's physician) asked me to stay on at St. Thomas' as his houseman, but I declined. A new start in a new country was what our young family needed.

Canada was our destination and on December 23, 1955, Lisa, Wilson, and I set sail from Southampton on the SS America for New York, and then onto Montreal.

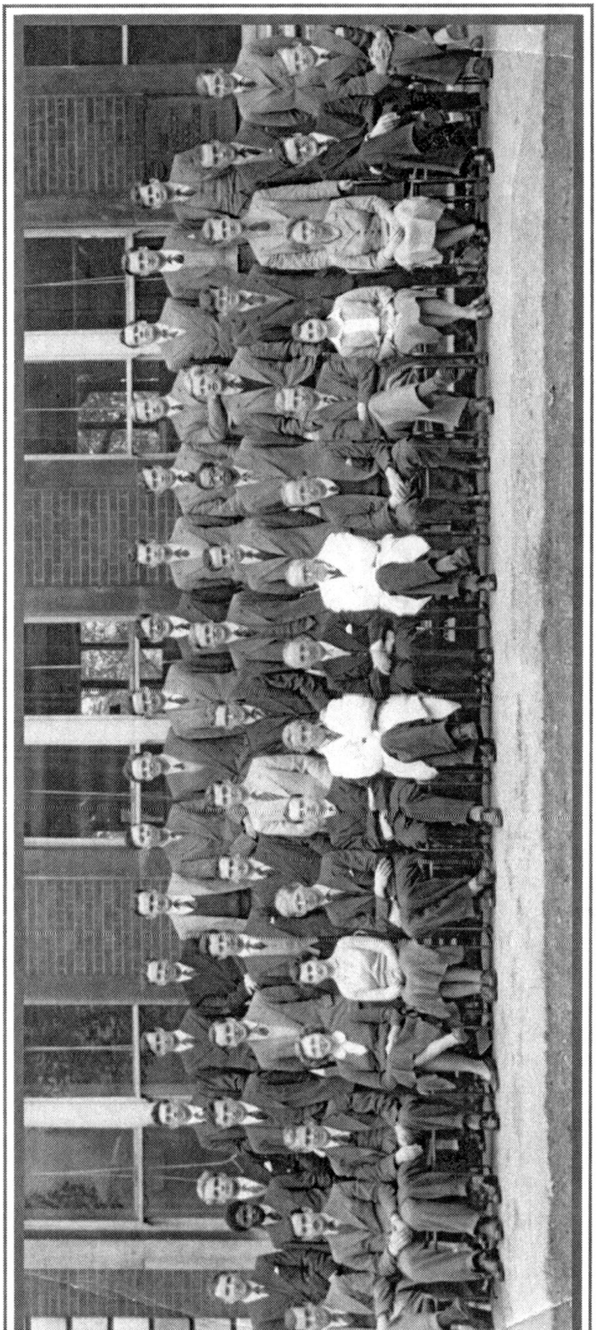

Class Photo, 1955

Montreal

- 1955 -

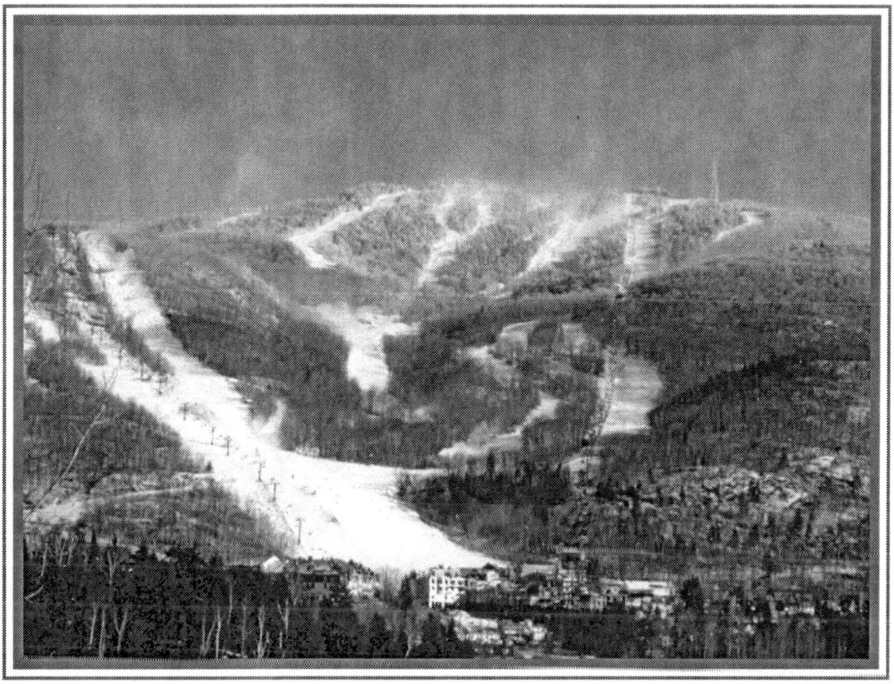

Mont Tremblant

December, 1955. The voyage from Southampton to New York City was an extremely rough crossing. More than half of the passengers were seasick, and we saw little of each other for most of the journey.

Wilson was barely 18 months, and fared amazingly well. As we were onboard for Christmas, the captain held a Christmas party for the children. Wilson received a small model of a locomotive train. By pressing a button, a voice was heard. "Tootle is a locomotive train, and as far as anyone can tell, Tootle is doing very well." That crossing was over fifty-five years ago.

The S.S. America arrived on time in New York, and we stayed overnight in a luxurious penthouse on Fifth Avenue. The weather in New York was clear, but cold. What I remember most about New York was the sight of those incredible skyscrapers, especially at night when the city was illuminated by a million lights. I had never seen a building higher than fifteen stories.

We caught the train to Montréal on the following morning, enjoying the brief journey along the way. The sights and sounds of this new country were exhilarating.

At the Windsor Station in Montreal, Dr. Robert Ash, the Medical Superintendent of Queen Elizabeth Hospital (the old homeopathic hospital of Montreal) was there to meet us. The weather was subzero fahrenheit, and we were inadequately dressed. Fingers, toes, nose, and ears were freezing, and we were unprepared for this type of bitter cold. In heaven's name, what have we come to? I could not help but wonder if leaving England was such a good idea.

Driving along Sherbrooke Street with dirty snow on the sidewalks and leafless trees was not what I had envisioned. Montréal in the winter is bleak, people tend to retire indoors for the most part, and when they do venture out they are well bundled up and almost unrecognizable.

We would come to realize that Montréal in the summer is a very different place—a vibrant city with tree-lined streets, sidewalk cafés, and great restaurants. It is a fun city, rightly called the "Paris of North America."

Montreal is actually an island in the St. Lawrence River. It took me several years to realize this! In order to get to the mainland, one has to cross one of several bridges.

The American border is barely sixty miles away from Montreal, and can be reached by car within a little over an hour. Plattsburgh and Burlington are the two largest cities from Montreal. They are close to the American border, and people periodically visit to buy American goods, cheaper.

We found accommodation at 5679 Prudomme Avenue, an absolute dump in NDG (Notre Dame de Grace), but quite near the hospital. The rent for our one-bedroom, sub-basement furnished apartment was eighty dollars a month, including heating. I recall the tenant who lived above us periodically throwing empty beer bottles out the window in his drunken state.

My parents were no longer helping us financially. We were on our own. My paycheck was only $150 a month and Lisa took a job for $200 a month, working four hours a day. Wilson stayed in the single interns' quarters while we both worked.

There were seven interns, two women and five men—from all over the world: Greece, Finland, Columbia, United States, and Canada. They were a great group. We were all broke, but had much fun during our internship year.

Penny was an intern who taught me how to tie knots using forceps (instrument tie). Because of my dyslexia, I was unable to tie knots any other way. The reef knot ties left over right, right over left. Or is it the other way around? I take back any unpleasant things I have said about women doctors! Penny was not only competent, but pretty and sexy (and married!)

Horatio was an intern from Colombia. He was so extremely homesick, and none of us could comfort him. After a few weeks, he abandoned his studies and flew back home.

Training at the Queen Elizabeth Hospital was excellent. After one year of rotating internship (three-month stints of obstetrics, gynecology, surgery, medicine and pediatrics), I felt I was ready to go into the big wide world and practice medicine.

The big advantage of interning in a hospital with no residents is that it is our call. There are no residents overseeing the doctor, which placed a great deal of responsibility on us. While we could always phone the staff man on call and he would readily come in if necessary, we tried to do this as little as possible.

Ambulance calls with a "one eyed" ambulance driver, Percy, were often frightening. Racing through red lights with sirens blaring was a major adrenaline rush and totally unnecessary! Taking stretchers up the outside winding metallic stairs, slippery and hard to reach top floors of duplexes in winter was difficult and dangerous.

At the end of our rotating internship year, we took the LMCC examination (Licentiate of the Medical Council of Canada). This license gave us the ability to practice anywhere in Canada except Quebec, Ontario, and British Columbia, unless we were a Canadian citizen (citizenship took five years to obtain).

Dr. Robert Ash, Professor of Anesthesiology at McGill, invited me to stay on in Québec. He "gave" me a homeopathic license, which allowed me to practice medicine in Quebec as a non-Canadian. Dr. Ash recommended I read several books on homeopathy from the hospital library. Read books? I had not read a book in my life!

This offer by Dr. Ash was a stroke of luck, as I was still a South African citizen. The license cost five dollars a year, signed by the Lieutenant Governor of the Province of Quebec. Another good example of the old boy grapevine, as Dr. Ash and my dad were good friends!

The LMCC exam was both written and oral. Dr. George Moore was one of my examiners in Obstetrics and Gynecology. He said, "Dr. Whyte, please give me all the indications for performing a hysterectomy." I gave him every single indication, having obtained my Cambridge degree only a year previously.

"No, doctor, you've left out a very important indication."

"Pray, what is that?"

"The quick, remunerative hysterectomy," he said.

This was a joke, of course, but in reality many hysterectomies have been performed unnecessarily.

For the next six months I did a "locum tenans" (hold the fort) for a doctor who was studying for a specialist degree in Cardiology. It was my first real experience in general practice.

One of my very first patients was Cleveland McDougal, a lean, lanky executive who came to me suffering from dipsomania, an interesting but not too common manifestation of alcoholism. An individual with this problem can go for lengthy periods without taking any alcohol, but when they do drink, they drink themselves into oblivion (a type of binge drinking).

I was determined to turn Cleveland into a social drinker. "You can have two drinks on any social occasion, but only two. No more."

For the first month, it seemed I had a social drinker. Such a clever doctor was I! I complimented Mr. McDougal on his successful sobriety. But alas, success was short-lived. Cleveland soon went on a colossal bender, fell down, and received a concussion with skull fracture. He was taken to Montreal General Hospital in delirium tremens.

McDougal was incontinent and had to be catheterized with an indwelling Foley catheter (a sterile rubber tube placed in the bladder and kept in place by a little balloon filled with water). Cleveland successfully managed to pull this out, a most traumatic undertaking!

I had learned a valuable lesson—that the treatment of alcoholism begins with abstinence—complete and total abstinence. Few alcoholics can attain abstinence on their own and need outside help and support such as that received in Alcoholics Anonymous.

Soon after his discharge from hospital, I phoned Cleveland and said, "Old chap, I have made a tremendous mistake.

You cannot do this on your own. It is blatantly obvious that my treatment was not only useless, but also dangerous. Please, go to an AA meeting. There are meetings all over town, morning, noon, and night. You will soon find a group that you feel comfortable with and, if you will take my humble suggestion, keep going back."

I went with McDougal to his first A. A. meeting. An incredibly friendly bunch of people greeted us at the door. McDougal never looked back, and has remained my patient and friend for many years.

For a couple of years, I worked part-time in the medical department of Alcan. There, I met the Medical Director, Dr. Douglas Watson, a great chap. Many of Alcan's senior executives were having two or three "bird bath martinis" for lunch, and their productivity would fall to zero in the afternoon. Their rehabilitation was important to the company, as many of these men had years of valuable experience which the company did not wish to loose.

There was a psychiatrist at the Veterans Hospital who was considered a "guru" in the treatment of alcoholism. I phoned him, asking for his secret. His response? "Do your level best to persuade the alcoholic to go to AA and stay there!"

Alanon is also an incredible organization for the families of alcoholics. Never forget that alcoholism is a family disease. The alcoholic is in trouble with the booze, and the spouses and family are in trouble with the boozer.

Living with an alcoholic can be absolute hell, and it is so important for the families of alcoholics to get help for themselves. Alanon is a magnificent support group.

Alcoholism is a complex, equal opportunity disease.

Pubs, palaces, and prisons—alcoholics come from every strata of society. Denial is the big reason why it is so difficult, if not impossible, for the alcoholic to make a self-diagnosis!

Keep in mind, a newcomer to AA may have to go to several different meetings before finding a compatible group.

Plain and simple, alcoholism is a disease. If left untreated, it will progress. Dementia, detention in jail or a hospital, and even death can be the result of this deceptive disease. How many times has an alcoholic told the spouse, "I'll never drink again," only to go on and drink again? For an alcoholic, all the willpower in the world will not bring sobriety.

Alcohol is perhaps the third leading cause of death. Fatal automobile and pedestrian accidents and the ravages of this substance on every organ of the body is often responsible.

"My name is Johnny, or Susan, and I am an alcoholic" (and sincerely mean it) in an AA meeting may be a humiliating confession, but it can also be the first essential step to a sober life.

Recovery is a lifelong process, and the alcoholic must really understand that there is no way possible to return to social drinking. Abstinence, abstinence, and abstinence is but the beginning in the treatment of alcoholism.

Many years ago, someone wrote these words:

We drank for happiness, and became unhappy;
We drank for joy, and became miserable;
We drank for sociability, and became argumentative;
We drank for sophistication, and became obnoxious;
We drank for friendship, and made enemies;
We drank for sleep, and awakened without rest;
We drank for strength, and felt weak;
We drank medicinally, and acquired health problems;
We drank for relaxation, and got the shakes;
We drank for bravery, and became afraid;
We drank for confidence, and became doubtful;
We drank to make conversation easier, and slurred our speech;
We drank to feel heavenly, and felt like hell;
We drank to forget, and were ever haunted;
We drank for freedom, and became slaves;
We drank to erase problems, and saw them multiply;
We drank to cope with life, and invited death.

Always remember, the alcoholic drinks primarily because he or she is in denial and has the DISEASE of alcoholism, affecting body, mind, and spirit.

On June 23, 1957 our daughter Julie was born. Quite frankly, I did not expect a daughter as my whole family was inundated with boys.

Julie was a chubby little thing and soon became the apple of my eye. She grew up to be a beautiful young woman. In her twenties she would be very fortunate to escape from a drug cartel in the Colombian jungle—an adventure quite remarkable, and I've always felt would be the makings of a great movie.

Lisa and I moved our family to Lakeshore, a lovely suburb on the

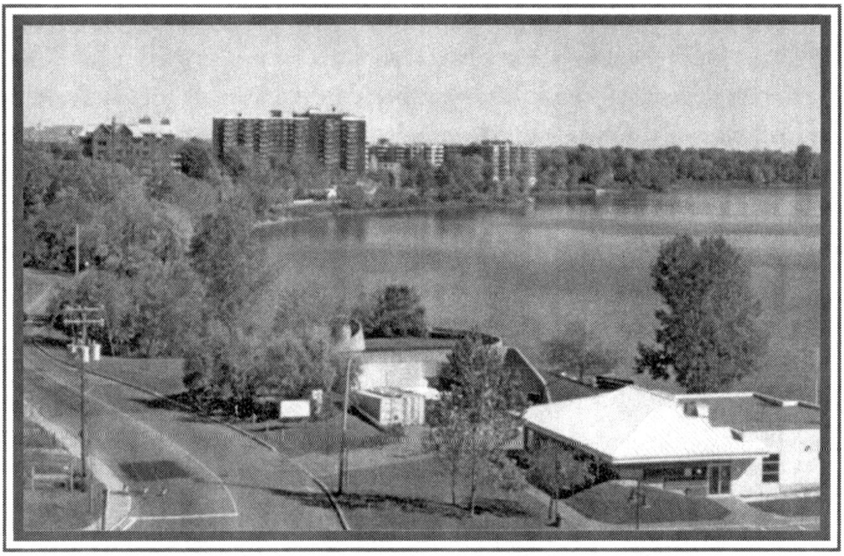

Lovely Lake Shore, West Island of Montreal

West Island of Montreal. It had a young, growing community, and was an ideal place to start my family practice.

The Royal Bank of Canada loaned me the money for a down payment on our home ($18,500). I also purchased a 1955 Chevrolet Biscayne for $1,500 on borrowed money.

My office was on the ground floor of our split-level home, with a separate entrance for patients, and on May 1, 1958 I put up my shingle and waited for the telephone to ring!

Alcan and Canadair had medical departments and, in my early days of practice I worked for them several hours a week. This income allowed me to build up my general practice.

At Canadair, I once did a pre-employment examination for a British DFC air ace who was to be employed as a senior test pilot. He was an overweight man in his late forties, and reeked of tobacco. On examination, I found uncontrolled high blood pressure and severe bronchitis and emphysema. I submitted an unfavorable report, but Canadair was apparently hell-bent to employ him anyway and he was accepted. Barely a month later, the man dropped dead at his desk.

Another patient, Frank Booth, was a pilot at Canadair. He took me up in one of their newest test planes—an exhilarating experience! What I remember most profoundly about the Booths was their son, Jerry. Jerry was left one cold Christmas morning on their front door step in a shoe box. Unable to trace his parents, the Booths adopted him and gave him a wonderful loving home. This scenario would appear to have come directly out of a Charles Dickens' novel!

About four-thirty one afternoon, a man came to me for a life insurance examination. He had just completed flying lessons at Canadair. After the examination, he asked me if I would like to go for a ride with him in his new single engine plane. I thanked him, but declined, telling him that after he had done a thousand successful takeoffs and landings, I would reconsider!

A week later, the man's plane crashed. People observing the crash felt this could well be a suicide, as he made no corrective maneuvers and crashed straight into the ground. Whether the life insurance company ever paid I do not know, but whenever I drove past his home at 369 Fields Boulevard, I thanked my lucky stars!

Building a new medical practice takes much time and hard work. I worked nights and weekends, and took calls for other doctors.

In retrospect, I did not realize just how depressed Lisa had become. We had two small children and, in addition, she was helping me run my office. She missed England.

Our sex life left a lot to be desired, and we never discussed things. Lisa had several sessions with a psychiatrist, Dr. McIntyre, but I was never included in any family counseling.

By the summer of 1961, I was doing well enough in practice to be able to rent a lovely log cabin on Lac Masson Ste. Marguerite in the Laurentian Mountains for the summer months.

Ste. Marguerite is an hour's drive from Montreal, and I commuted back and forth to visit Lisa and the kids at the cabin on Wednesday afternoons and on weekends when I was not on call.

The Laurentian Mountains are some of the oldest in the world, and the whole area has many beautiful lakes. Many who live in the area sometimes commuted to work in Montréal each day, as it is an easy drive on a superhighway.

There are some wonderful ski resorts in the Laurentians. It is a most popular area for families to spend summer holidays, and in the winter skiers cannot wait to hit the slopes after the first good snowfall! Mont Tremblant, Grey Rocks, and the Mont Gabriel Club are a few of the favorite skiing spots. In days of old, Mont Gabriel did not welcome Jews.

We were finding that Montréal and its environs were a wonderful place to work and play. Our rustic log cabin was right on the water, a fisherman's paradise, with large speckled and rainbow trout. In June, the black flies are a nuisance!

There were several families with children close by in cottages, and we made new friends. I especially enjoyed the tennis courts and found some good doubles players. One of these was Mario.

Mario was an excellent left-handed player. He had a beautiful Italian wife, Sophia, and four young boys ranging in age from five to twelve. As head of a large Swiss bank, Mario could take as much time off as he wished. It was rumored that Mario was a millionaire many times over, and also had a roving eye.

Lisa and I became close friends with Mario and Sophia. Our children also got on well and spent their days fishing, canoeing, and swimming. The fresh mountain air and break from the office was also good for Lisa, and her depression improved dramatically.

And so—practice was good, Lisa was happy, and my dad and I had completely reconciled. In 1962, we bought a lovely new home very close to the water on the Lakeshore. It was a happy time for us. But alas—it would not last long.

The whole family went to South Africa in the summer of 1962 to visit my parents and show off Julie and Wilson. It had been ten years since my last visit to South Africa. Things had changed, but the whites were still living in the lap of luxury!

The children learned to ride horses at a riding school owned by a very masculine looking woman named Mrs. Biggs. We visited the Kruger National Park, a wild game park the size of England. Elephants, lions, leopards—you name it—were all there in their natural habitat. The kids enjoyed their visit to South Africa to see their South African Granny and Grandpa for the first time, and the wild animals, of course!

On our return journey, Lisa and the kids stopped over in England for a month to visit her parents and let the English grandparents meet Wilson, now seven, and Julie, age five.

After their visit in England, the family returned to Montréal with a golden retriever, "Shona," a beautiful dog. Shona was with us for the next fourteen years. I had really wanted a Dandie Dinmont, but Lisa felt they were too yappy. Terriers do tend to bark a lot.

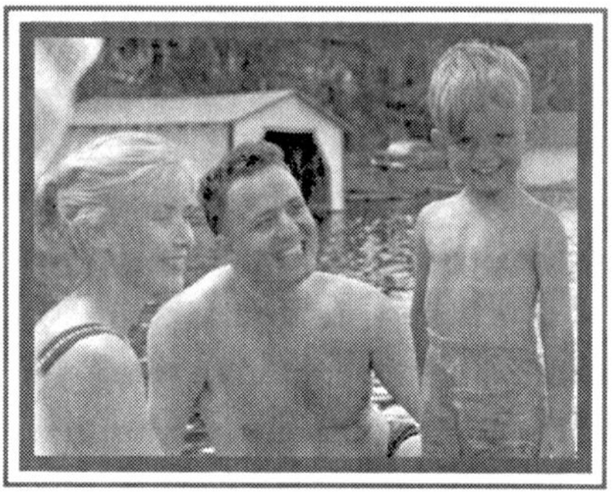

Lisa, Ian, and Wilson
Cambridge. "The Cuckold."

While in England, Lisa visited our old friend Derek, who had been a member of the St. Thomas' camera club. He was now a family doctor practicing in Knightsbridge. Derek gave Lisa some magazines featuring some of Steve's beautiful black-and-white nude photographs.

When Lisa returned from England, she seemed like a different person. No longer depressed, and loving our home, Lisa started to go shopping several times a week. Mrs. Watson, an elderly patient of mine, often babysat.

Mrs. Watson once confided in me that her married daughter was having an affair and she covered for her daughter, Marguerite, pretending to the husband that they were having lunch in town. Marguerite had been married for ten years to a rat-like little man, a patient of mine who was a complete Mr. Dullsville.

During this time, I was so preoccupied with my practice that I failed to notice that Lisa seldom came home with parcels. Not for one moment did I suspect that she, too, might be having an affair. To my dyslexic mind, night was the time for lovemaking. Just how stupid could I be?

During the next two years, Lisa developed a passion for "shopping."

In the meantime, I was building one of the largest and most successful practices on the Lakeshore. I loved my practice and really cared for my patients, and they seemed to like and trust me as well. Family practice can be a most rewarding branch of medicine.

I could write a book on my interactions with patients, but it would take a lifetime. Following are a few anecdotes you may find interesting, funny, perhaps strange, or even nasty.

There was an old widowed nursery school teacher, a Miss Grant, who would come every fall for an annual flu shot. After a few pleasantries, and a lengthy discussion of her cat's recent illness, I gave the flu shot. On one occasion, just as she was about to leave the office, she said, "Oh doctor, I think I might have some hemorrhoids. Would you mind taking a look?" "By all means, Miss Grant, just remove your bloomers."

I was examining Miss Grant's nether regions with a gloved hand when, at that split second, in walked my pretty nurse, Katy. Katy took one look and quickly said, "Please, Doctor, remind me never to come to you for a flu shot!"

Stanley was a patient who came to me with a unique and unusual complaint. He was in his early forties, a charming, good-looking man, and always immaculately dressed. He said, "Doctor, I don't want you to think any the less of me, but I have a hobby which involves the seduction of married women."

Not flinching, I asked him to tell me more, and in the next twenty minutes he told me the following story almost verbatim.

"Approaching a good looking woman with trim figure, I always look for a wedding ring. It is important to make absolutely sure she is married. With my experience, I invariably can tell if the woman is likely to be a vulnerable candidate! Many women have husbands who are sexually inadequate."

He continued. "A beer, a steak, and a screw just will not cut it. Mr. Doubtfire, in the movie played by the American actor, Robin Williams, had said, "Brace yourself, Bridget." This was Mr. Doubtfire's pathetic idea of foreplay! Wine, dinner, and beautiful flowers—all are part of my own elaborate seduction plan. This may take some time, but time is on my side."

Stanley continued his story. "Many of these women have never been unfaithful since their marriage. This is all the more titillating! Gentle persuasion and firmness are the essential ingredients to a woman's psychological seduction.

Anticipation can be highly erotic and almost as exciting as the finale!

The climax, so to speak, takes place in a 5-star hotel, where I have my usual private suite booked. Nothing is hurried. During their high school years, many of these young women have smoked pot, and I always have some of the finest British Columbia Gold available. A joint and a delicious martini will invariably relax a woman's highest moral fiber. Watching another man's attractive wife slowly disrobe after a champagne lunch in my suite is exciting. With lengthy innovative foreplay, my ability to retard ejaculation indefinitely ensures uninhibited and abandoned sex.

Doctor, I find that married women are often capable of enjoying raw sex with a lover that they could never have with a husband. To savor a woman having multiple prolonged orgasms, feel the tight intermittent squeeze with each paroxysm of ecstasy, and be able to control and withhold one's own pleasure—this, doctor, gives me an incredible atavistic rush! Almost the culmination of the hunt!

After a brief rest and a cigarette, we continue making love, until my exhausted prey begs me to stop. Stop I will, but not before I make sure she climaxes several more times. It is only then that I will allow myself the long withheld, pent-up explosion.

Invariably the lady would love to repeat our rendezvous and, having her telephone number, I promise—but the game is over.

My modus operandi had never failed, until a few days ago. All was going splendidly, but suddenly my Ambassador would not rise to the occasion. Completely devastating! What is my problem, Doctor?" Stanley seemed to be finished with his story.

With a serious expression on my face betraying very mixed emotions of envy and admiration, I lied, "Stanley, this happens to everyone on occasion. The more you worry, the worse it gets. Just relax old man. Stop fretting."

Proceeding to examine his genitalia, I found a fine specimen of manhood. He was built like a stallion with two firm testicles slightly smaller than golf balls. "Stanley, there is absolutely nothing wrong with you." Reassurance from a trusted doctor works like magic!

All went well after our visit, and I am sure many a lovely lady found her way into Stanley's Ritz-Carlton suite, succumbing in wanton and bitter sweet surrender.

Having heard Stanley's story, I couldn't help but wonder how married women feel about living in lifelong single penile servitude? The sad part of Stanley's story is that he left his wife and two daughters, and fled to South Africa.

His wife loved Stanley, and never fully recovered. The last time I saw her—when I was doing a house call in the area—she had become a stooped over, gray little woman, going door-to-door selling Fuller brushes.

Jerry was eighteen when he came to my office complaining of a cough he had suffered with for a month. He was a husky young lad and looked like a football player. There was nothing significant in his history.

My examinations were always thorough as I never want to overlook anything—ears, nose, throat, heart, lungs, abdomen, and testicles. You may think it strange that a patient coming in for a cough exam gets his testicles examined, but Jerry had a lump in his right testicle the size of a baseball.

"Jerry, why didn't you tell me about this?"

He responded by saying, "But it doesn't hurt, doctor." (Much like the familiar "painless lump" in breast cancer.)

Jerry's chest x-ray revealed "cannonball secondaries" from a carcinoma of the testicle—the reason for his cough!

I sent Jerry to an oncologist, Dr. John Tonkin. The testicle was removed, and the pathology revealed the same type of cancer Lance Armstrong had. This uncommon type of cancer is highly treatable with chemotherapy and testicle removal.

The secondry cancers in Jerry's chest disappeared. Jerry eventually got married, but there would be no children.

Recently, forty years later, I by chance met Jerry's aunt in an elevator and asked her how Jerry was doing. She said he had just turned fifty-eight, and was in the process of a divorce.

Bruce was an extremely wealthy patient, an alcoholic. He was not looking for help with his drinking, but came to my office with this story.

He had flown to San Francisco, rented a large sailboat and crew, and employed the services of several lovely women. After a week on the sailboat he returned to Montreal, having absolutely no memory of the whole trip. Only when his credit card statement came in was he able to tell where he had been.

This condition is called alcoholic global amnesia. To use the vernacular—major memory blackout (blanks).

Bruce's alcoholism resulted in his early death. Remember the three D's—detention, delirium and death. It is one nasty disease affecting family, friends, work, and everything else.

The Rentons were a lovely family living on the Lakeshore. Donald worked for a large pharmaceutical company. He worked hard all his life and decided to retire when he turned fifty-three. It was a life ambition to take his family on a world cruise, but tragedy struck and he died shortly before reaching fifty-three. Always a heavy smoker, Bruce had suffered a fatal heart attack.

Dorothy Renton had called me in my office when he collapsed, and I immediately made a house call. It was sudden death, with absolutely no chance of resuscitation. This was long before defibrillators and, even if one had been available, it could not have helped poor Don. He was dead. When it is one's time to go this is the best way, but a totally unexpected happening like this is devastating to the family.

As I was trying to console Dorothy, who was weeping uncontrollably, their drunken neighbor, Bernie, walked in. Bernie was also a patient of mine. He had reached the bottom of the barrel with his alcoholism and would drink anything, including aftershave lotion.

We had not heard Bernie come in the front door, which was ajar. Completely inebriated, he staggered up to the bedroom and fell across the bed where Don lay. Strange bedfellows, in a most macabre scene.

It took a second to realize what had happened, and then I pushed him off the bed and onto the floor. He lay there on the floor in a semi-coma, mumbling words of condolences. With great difficulty, Dorothy and I finally got him out of their home.

Once an extremely successful businessman, Bernie died just six months later from cirrhosis of the liver, a direct result of chronic alcoholism.

A young woman in her early twenties came to visit me at the office, looking very depressed. She had two small boys, ages two and three. Without wasting any time, she asked me, "How often do you think a married couple should have sexual relations?"

Taken by surprise at this unheralded question, my answer was, "It depends on a variety of things. For instance, if you are on vacation you might have more frequent sexual relations than at other times." I was hedging, trying to feel her out a bit.

She asked, "What about five times?" I thought she was referring to five times a week. "Well, considering your age, that does not sound unreasonable." "No, doctor, you misunderstand, I mean five times a night, every night." By now she was crying.

This completely took me off guard. I was dumbfounded. "Young lady, that strikes me as grossly abnormal!"

"Well, this is exactly what is happening, and I am completely exhausted!" Her husband, Angus, was a lean, lanky Scotsman with a rapacious sexual appetite.

His brother was the same! He took a date to dinner, and afterwards had sexual activity. That same evening, he would pick up a second date and do the same thing all over again. (Of all my years in medical practice, this incredible sexual gold medal marathon performer stands out vividly in my memory.)

To cut a long story short, the distraught young wife had a suicide attempt and, shortly thereafter, they divorced.

Sexual appetites and performances vary tremendously. I have made an observation, without any medical foundation, that lean wiry men are often the most horny! I later confirmed this observation in my own mind when Lisa ran off with such an individual. Granted, he was filthy rich as well!

The mother of one of my patients, Mrs. Watson stormed into my office one day in anger. "You had no right to give Dr. Bill Benjamin my daughter's telephone number," she said. I had absolutely no idea what Mrs. Watson was talking about!

Sylvia, her daughter, was an attractive nineteen-year-old student at Sir George Williams College in Montréal. I did not know a Dr. Bill Benjamin, but if I had, I would certainly not have given him a patient's telephone number.

What may have happened is that the imposter could have placed a random telephone call, to which Sylvia happened to answer. Or perhaps he knew her from Sir George Williams College. He identified himself as "Dr. Bill Benjamin" and said he had been given her phone number by her family doctor. To this, Sylvia probably replied with, "Oh! You mean Dr. Whyte"—thus giving my name away.

"Dr. Benjamin" then asked Sylvia to give him her name to make sure he was speaking to the right person. In doing so, she gave her own name away!

The bogus Dr. Benjamin likely said he was conducting a sexual survey on female students. Would Sylvia be prepared to participate? Sylvia, thinking all was on the up and up, readily agreed.

The questions, as you can imagine, were very personal. "How often do you have sexual relations?" "How often do you masturbate?" "How do you masturbate?" "What do you think about when you masturbate?" And so on, and so forth.

These telephone conversations went on for several weeks. Finally, Mrs. Watson overheard some of Sylvia's conversation, answers to the questions. The understandably furious mother then paid a visit to my office.

A wiretap was placed on the Watson's telephone. It was ultimately discovered that "Dr. Bill Benjamin" was calling from Sir George Williams College. Unfortunately, the wiretap could go no further than the college switchboard.

The calls abruptly stopped, but not until after Dr. Bill Benjamin received a well-deserved scathing tongue lashing from Mrs. Watson. (Of course, this story is a classic example of the extent to which sexual perverts will go.)

A young husband came to my office with a tablet he found in his wife's handbag. He wanted my confirmation that this was the birth control pill. It was the pill. Since he was sterile, he became highly suspicious and had his wife followed. Sure enough, there was hanky-panky going on.

They went for marriage counseling. She was always immaculately dressed. After their session, she drove off to a motel to meet her lover! Prognosis poor!

Another heartbroken woman came to my office. Her husband of fourteen years, a schoolteacher, had confessed to her that he was homosexual and that he had decided to leave her and her two teenage daughters for a young man.

In yet another situation, a Miss Universe competition was taking place in Montréal. A participant, Miss Scandinavia, was brought to me by a friend. They wanted me to confirm a pregnancy.

Miss Scandinavia was a tall beautiful brunette in her early twenties. After repeating the pregnancy test twice and performing a pelvic examination, there was no doubt she was about eight to ten weeks pregnant. The two women left my office distraught.

Abortions were illegal in Montréal at that time. A druggist friend later informed me that the two women had located an abortionist, but would do the job only if Miss Scandinavia agreed to spend the night with him in addition to his five hundred dollar fee! Here we have another example of a sexual pervert, with the added fraud.

Recently I heard from the woman who brought the pregnant Miss Scandinavia to my office. She told me that Miss Scandinavia returned to her country where she married and started a family.

Peggy was a patient who came to me with a strange problem. Her husband always insisted that whenever she leaves home she must first insert a glass test tube into her vagina. Perversion once again, and a very ridiculous request without any logic whatsoever! I removed the test tube, and told Peggy to stop such dangerous practice immediately.

A married couple came to my office saying that they had found their teenage son and daughter having sex. What should they do?

I once examined a young married woman, Julia, for her annual physical. While performing a pap test, she had a prolonged orgasm. Julia was most embarrassed, and when it was over apologized profusely. Reassuring her, I told her not to give it a second thought, as this was not uncommon. A monumental white lie!

Some women do fantasize about having sex with their physician, so it is essential for doctors to have a nurse present at all times when performing any such exam, and that includes exam of breasts.

Brian was a young McGill student who, together with a group of researchers, worked one summer in the Arctic Circle. It was night and they were all asleep in their tent when a huge polar bear broke in. The little dog with them in the tent immediately started barking furiously. The starving beast attacked Brian with his massive claws, almost pulling off an ear. Thanks to the little dog's early barking, one of the researchers managed to kill the bear with a shotgun but not before it had killed the little dog.

They bandaged up Brian's head, preserving his ear, and transported him by air back to the Lakeshore General Hospital, where I was on duty. His face was unrecognizable, and his ear literally hung by a thread. Dr. Alfonzo Cigarre, a brilliant plastic surgeon, performed plastic surgery. He managed to reattach the ear, preserving the facial nerve and thus avoiding a hideous facial deformity.

An autopsy on the bear revealed seaweed in its stomach. Apparently a polar bear will only eat seaweed if it is starving. Brian came to me for follow-up a week later and told me this amusing story:

When checking in at the Lakeshore General Hospital follow-up clinic, the woman at the desk asked Brian the reason for his visit. He said, "I was mauled by a polar bear." Without looking up, the woman casually asked, "Anything else?"

In the good old days, one could spend a bit of time with patients, and visit. Many of my patients became good friends, and I considered myself privileged to look after them.

At Christmastime, we decorated my office and had a small Christmas tree. Patients sent Christmas cards, wrote kind thank-you notes, and frequently brought homemade goodies.

One Christmas, Mrs. Polly Sansom brought me a box of delicious shortbread made from her mother's recipe. I telephoned Mrs. Sansom just recently (we had not spoken or seen each other in over thirty years) to get her permission to share with you her mother's shortbread recipe. She said I was more than welcome to let my readers have it.

Even if you may not like my book, I can absolutely guarantee that this old and closely guarded secret family recipe is well worth the price of the book! Follow the recipe instructions carefully.

Mrs. Tyne Alcorn's (1887-1985) Family Secret delicious shortbread recipe.

Batter:
1 pound very soft butter
3-3-1/2 c. flour (more if needed)
Heat oven to 300 degrees. Slowly mix the flour with the butter until it forms a soft but not sticky dough. On a flour board, pat the dough until it is 1/2 inch thick (or slightly less).

Using a round cutter (1-1/2 inch in diameter), cut the cookies and place them on a cookie sheet. Bake for 25 to 30 minutes, or until slightly golden. Remove and cool. Since there is no sugar in the cookies, they can be frosted and topped with red or green candied cherries.

Icing:
1/4 c. butter
2-1/2 c. icing sugar
3-4 T. milk or cream

Cream butter and gradually add icing sugar and cream to make spreading consistency. Add more sugar or cream, as necessary. After icing cookies, top with pieces of cherry.

It is difficult to pinpoint exactly when Lisa's drinking began to escalate. When we originally met, she drank very little. But escalate it did, and with it came many behavioral problems.

We both saw psychiatrists (a man and wife team) on several occasions, but they were unable to help and simply told me to take all alcohol out of the house! Absolutely useless advice.

Sex life had become almost nonexistent, and one morning before work she caught me masturbating. Immediately she said, "Don't stop," and rolled over and went back to sleep. I was chagrined and very embarrassed.

Putting on my shoes as I sat on our bed, I must have woken her. She angrily said, "Never put your shoes on while sitting on the side of the bed while I am trying to sleep!"

Lisa had been drinking just before leaving our home one morning and had consumed six ounces of vodka. She was involved in a serious auto accident on the TransCanada Highway, and cited in a six-car pileup after she ran into the back of a stationary car at a red light.

In the following weeks, I monitored her vodka consumption by marking the bottle. This is done by turning the bottle upside down, leaving a very tiny mark at the top of the fluid level. This way, when the bottle is turned correct way up, no mark is visible.

We had invited three couples to have dinner with us one Friday evening. The couples arrived at six p.m., but no Lisa. She was presumably still shopping. The babysitter, Mrs. Watson, had left at five p.m.

Suddenly, Lisa arrived home at six thirty, flushed, blaming the traffic. Hurriedly, she ran upstairs to our bedroom. I was right behind her and saw her throw a white circular object into our metallic clothes basket. It made a very audible sound. Looking into the clothes basket, I found her plastic diaphragm case containing a moist diaphragm. No explanation was offered and since we had dinner guests, I did not pursue the subject.

This was my first indication of Lisa's adultery. I did not have the remotest idea who her lover could be, and so I silently named him "Mr. X." The detectives I employed were two French Canadians, Caduc and Desrosier. They patiently waited for Lisa to leave home but, unfortunately, following her was difficult. She drove at such high speed around the dorval circle in her blue Karmen Ghia, they lost her.

In Canada at that time, to get a divorce one must have unequivocal adultery evidence. So, what to do? The solution was quite simple. Check the mileage on her odometer, which consistently read eighteen miles from our home (nine miles there, and nine miles back). A radius of nine miles gave two possible areas where Lisa "went shopping"—one was on the Upper Lachine Road, and one very near Canadair.

The Upper Lachine Road motel drew a blank, but the Motel Pierre quite near Canadair proved to be where the mysterious Mr. X and Lisa had been meeting for well over two years.

Surveillance of Motel Pierre regularly showed her blue car parked outside the executive suite. The cleaning lady was bribed a hundred dollars to borrow the key, which was then duplicated.

On September 23, I received a call from the detectives saying they had just seen Mr. X and Lisa enter their love nest. My office was fully booked and I was in the middle of examining a patient. I asked the detective if I could finish my examination, but he said, "No, come immediately. How long do you think it takes, Doc?"

I told my new secretary (it was her first day on the job) that I had an emergency, and then raced off to the motel.

Within seconds of my arrival, the detectives opened the door—and there Lisa and her lover. Our entry must have coincided with a mutual orgasm, as I had never heard Lisa make such anguished cries!

It took several seconds for them to realize there were three other people in the room. Mr. X—the mysterious lover—was none other than Mario, my tennis friend from Ste. Marguerite. He was lying on his back, with Lisa straddling him. Both were naked except for Mario, who was wearing a pair of bright blue socks. Lisa's bra was lying on the floor, and the pillows and bed sheets were in disarray.

The detectives quickly took pictures, which would later be used in court as evidence of adultery.

Lisa's outcry after things had subsided was, "What the hell are you doing here?" I felt this was quite a strange question and responded, "Pray, what the hell are You doing here?"

In a flash, my whole world came crashing down—our wedding in the little church outside Amersham, the birth of our kids, and all the happy times I thought we had. Any man or woman who has been through this experience knows exactly what I am talking about. It is a crushing blow to one's ego, and devastatingly painful.

Mario's wife knew nothing of the affair, and Mario was a very worried man. He came to my office the next morning, begging me to take Lisa back. That afternoon, the children and I went to the Queen Elizabeth Hotel to pick up their mummy. I paid for the hotel room—which came with a large booze bill!

Lisa promised me that the affair was over and that she would never see Mario again. By taking her home, I had condoned Lisa's adultery, destroying all my divorce evidence.

Two months later, Lisa and Mario were back in bed.

This time, following her was much more difficult. She drove to a certain place, parked her car, and then took a taxi to Mario's mother's apartment.

She did not see me follow her, so I was able to tell the detectives where the new hideout was. As he pocketed another five hundred dollars, Detective Caduc asked, "When are you ever going to learn, Doc?"

The marriage was over, and Lisa had temporary custody of the children. Mario left his wife and four children, and moved in with Lisa.

Our home on the Lakeshore was sold for a good deal less than I paid for it, and I moved into an apartment beneath my office. The day the real estate agent put a "sold" sign on our front lawn, Wilson (now seven) cried and asked, "Daddy, I love this house, why are you selling it?"

The only things I was able to salvage from our breakup were two beautiful watercolors of young Pondo African Tribe women with their colorful blankets, a dresser, and a mattress (with an inscription, "Enchanted Nights." What irony.

Mario's wife, Sofia, was devastated when she discovered what had been going on for so long. It appears to be a well-known fact that the spouse is usually the last one to know. After an almost successful suicide attempt, Sophia was admitted to the psychiatric unit of the Boswell Memorial hospital. While there, Sofia met an extremely good-looking psychiatrist by the name of Alan.

It gets a little complicated here! Alan moved to Vermont. Since her custody court order prevented her from taking the four boys to Vermont, Sophia and Alan broke up temporarily.

Fairly soon thereafter, Sofia met Lawrence, an industrial tycoon, and moved in with him. It seemed that Sophia had found the man of her dreams. However, just a few days before the marriage, Lawrence informed Sofia that he intended to leave all of his money to his six children from previous marriages. Heartbroken, Sophia went back to Alan who was still living in Vermont!

Alan and Sofia moved to Hawaii taking Keith, her youngest, who was now old enough to accompany them.

Finally, Sofia discovered that the good-looking psychiatrist, Alan, was bisexual with a preference for young men!

Meanwhile, Lisa and Mario had been living together. When Sofia told Mario that he was not Keith's father, Mario flew into a rage. He married Lisa the following week!

The marriage of Lisa and Mario was destined to wind up on the rocks. In the end, they were in and out of court seventeen times in one year!

"Oh, what tangled webs of woe we weave, when first we venture to deceive."—Sir Walter Scott (1771-1894)

Many years after our divorce, Lisa and I met for a visit over lunch. By then, she and Mario had divorced and I was happily married to Rosemary.

Lisa had recently been in an alcohol rehabilitation center in Stowe, Vermont. Her "significant other" was Barry, a part-time disc jockey and taxi driver whom she had met in rehab.

We lunched at the Green Lantern Tavern (Lanterna Verde), a wonderful place with great Italian food. Lisa ordered a bird bath vodka martini, and I a Molson Premium beer. The martini disappeared quickly, and she ordered another one. This was disappointing to witness as apparently rehab did her little good. Delicious pasta was accompanied by a bottle of Chateau la Garde '57, and then Lisa vented with a confessional to me noted below pretty much verbatim.

Quote. "Ian, I never told you any of this before, but I realized soon after our first date that you were a lousy fuck. During the ten years we were married, I never climaxed once. Each time you asked me if I had gone to the moon (had a climax), I said yes to appease you.

Before you, David was my boyfriend. If I had not gotten pregnant by you, I would have probably married him. David and I continued to see each other on occasion until you and I left for Canada.

Bertie Krantz also saw me on one occasion. When you were in hospital with Mono, we spent a long weekend together in Salisbury. Fairly soon after Wilson was born, I began seeing David again. You never suspected a thing—blissfully unaware.

When I started nude modeling for the camera club, I often had sex with Derek, Nicholas and Steve. (We had met Derek and Nick on a St. Thomas' ski trip at St. Antoine in Austria.)

You knew the camera club met at Steve's lovely home in Chelsea. The shoot would begin half an hour after cocktails. Steve would pour me two or three stiff Gin martinis over the course of the evening. After disrobing, the club members would photograph me in various poses with or without props.

Steve was not into group sex, but enjoyed photographing it. He and I would occasionally have sex in his mirrored bedroom, always alone.

What I did not know at the time was that Steve had state-of-the-art surveillance cameras in his bedroom. At his leisure, he could revisit all my oblivious, uninhibited sexual performances with him as well as with the other camera club youngsters!

Steve's favored pastime was watching these erotic films while sipping Harvey's Bristol Cream Sherry and smoking Black Russian Sobrani cigarettes.

Another of Steve's turn-on's was photographing "menage a trois"—Nick, Derek and myself in all sorts of erotic positions!

Many of Steve's superb black-and-white nude photographs appeared in English photographic journals and in a well-known, widely circulated magazine, "Men Only."

One day, Steve went out in his sailboat in the British Virgins, and never returned. Sad to say, neither Steve nor his sailboat were ever found.

The other thing I never told you, I got pregnant with Mario's child while you were in the Montreal General Hospital having nasal surgery. Neither Mario nor you ever knew. You later prescribed a medication called kevadon (thalidomide) for my early morning nausea.

Nobody knew of the devastating effects thalidomide could have on an unborn child. Ironically, it was an excellent antinauseant and a very good non-addicting sleep medication.

I insisted I did not want to have another child, and you had made arrangements with one of your gynecological buddies to do a D&C on the grounds that I was spontaneously aborting." End quote.

Lisa's confession ended with a description of Mario's sexual secret. He would climax quickly initially, she said, but from then on, using a breathing technique, perform like an Olympian! (Was she trying to rub salt into my wounds?)

Can you imagine the scenario had Lisa had gone forward with her pregnancy? Mario's child (unknown to both him and me) could have been born a thalidomide baby, without arms or legs.

I have no idea why Lisa felt the need to tell me all of this, but I have no reason to disbelieve her disturbing confessions "in veno veritas." Perhaps she felt this may be our last visit together. It was!

Lisa, my ex-wife who did not want thousands of dollars, but hundreds of thousands of dollars, died penniless with a breast malignancy a few years later at the age of fifty-nine. Our daughter, Julie, paid for her mother's funeral expenses. Lisa's ashes are buried in a cemetery outside Burlington.

I had no idea what a lousy fuck I was until I got this earful from Lisa. All the years I was married to her, I thought she was having silent climaxes when we made love! When I asked, she invariably said, "yes."

The other thing friends could not fathom was that Lisa returned home from shopping with no parcels. The fact that she ran around for two years during the day, and I never suspected anything, was probably due to my dyslexic brain.

So there you have the tale of a naive Cambridge PE cuckold, and the good reason the front of my memoirs contain an apology to all the women in my life who may have suffered from unrequited love.

In retrospect, it is not surprising that a woman who gets no sexual fulfillment from a husband or significant other, but is getting plenty of satisfying sex on the side, would regard sex with a premature ejaculator as a nuisance. An "intra-vaginal masturbation, of sorts!" The expression, "boom-bam, thankee, ma'am," did not come from thin air!

There are likely many women out there who are condemned to a lifetime of defective penile servitude. Reading between the sheets, I wonder how many women have perfected the art of faking orgasms? And the "orgasm oscar" goes to . . . Meg Ryan, in "Sleepless In Seattle!"

While the "PE condition" is not terribly unique, the misfortune of others gives one little comfort. Premature ejaculation is a dysfunction few men care to admit to as it is a most embarrassing and distressing subject. Yet, in today's more open society, talking it over with a trusted doctor may be helpful.

When I was a student at Cambridge University medical school, sex education was nonexistent. Had I had the opportunity then to read the works of Masters and Johnson (the initial phase of their 1957 to 1964 studies), I might have been ahead of the game!

To digress for a moment, I would like to return briefly to the subject of breast cancer.

In the United States in 2007, breast cancer was expected to cause over 40,000 deaths. Women have roughly a one-in-eight lifetime chance of developing invasive breast cancer. This figure has significantly increased since 1970, and many more younger women are becoming victims.

When my niece, Danielle, was twenty-eight, she developed breast cancer. Yet, Danielle is very much alive and well today, fifteen years later, thanks to early detection.

On June 23, 2007, I telephoned my daughter to wish her a happy fiftieth birthday. It was certainly not a happy day for her because she had recently been diagnosed with advanced breast cancer involving her left breast.

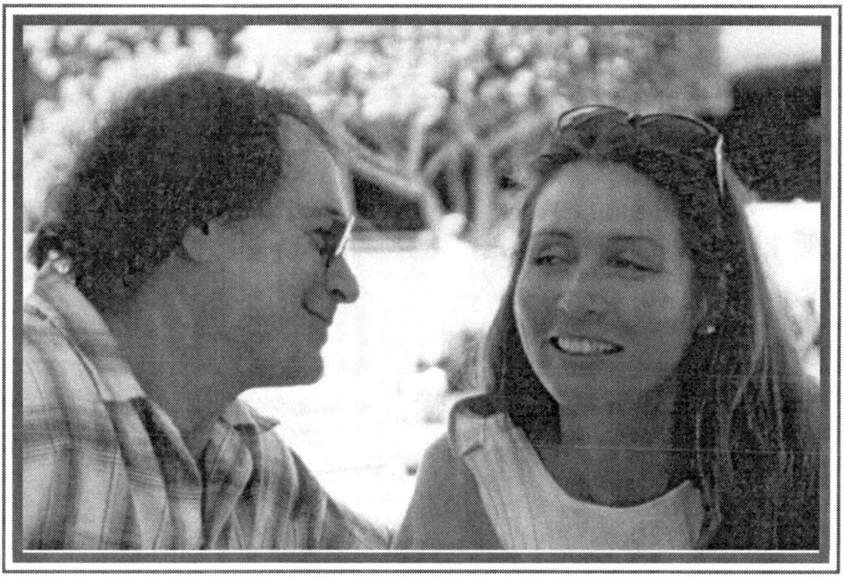

Julie and her husband, David

Julie religiously had mammograms taken every single year since the age of thirty-five. All were negative! Over the years, various doctors from very reputable hospitals had examined her annually. No lump palpated! She continued to complain that she felt "something was wrong in her left breast." One doctor told her it was all in her head!

> Scripps Memorial Hospital, La Jolla,
> La Jolla Radiology Medical Group. June 20 2007.
> Examination: Dynamic M.R. Mammography.
> MR Breast Bilateral. Very extensive involvement left breast,
> Invasive and itraductal carcinoma.
> Tumor Size: 15.7 cm by 4.3 cm

Julie's tumor was the size of a fist, a large fist, and it was not in her head!

Any time you feel there is something not right with your breast, do not be bamboozled by your M.D. Some doctors consistently play God. Unfortunately, their egos get in the way, and this prevents them from making a sound diagnosis.

Insist on a second opinion and an MRI mammography of the breasts, even if your regular mammograms were negative. A doctor's over-reliance on negative mammograms can be disastrous, and may well cost you your life.

Just remember, you have a much better chance of discovering early breast cancer by practicing regular, meticulous, breast self-examination. The reason for this is that your doctor may be concerned, if he gives you too lengthy and thorough an examination, that you will get the impression he is playing with your breasts and report him for inappropriate behavior.

I recently heard a report on television that self-examination of one's breasts is deemed unnecessary. I could not believe this criminal advice! Just wait and see the influx of undiagnosed breast cancer.

You have been warned. Please, do take heed. This warning and advice may just save your life.

When Lisa left me for Mario in 1963, my ego took a tremendous wallop and depression hit hard. At age thirty-three, I was a divorced man.

I lost a lot of weight, and sleeping was a problem. A psychiatrist I had been seeing put me on a drug called parstelin, a mixture of an anti-depressant (parnate) and phenothiazines (stelazine). This combination is no longer on the market. Within a few weeks, it had worked miracles. Soon, apart from a bruised ego, I was on the road to recovery.

I received custody of both my young children and placed them in boarding schools. The only time a man will receive custody of his children is when the wife is either an addict (alcoholic) or a paid prostitute.

Certainly, boarding school is not an ideal solution, but with a working father and a alcoholic mother, it seemed the best solution for the children at that time.

Julie was seven and Wilson was nine. They were good kids, and I visited them as often as my visitations permitted. Julie was the youngest boarder ever at Dawkins School for Girls. Both excellent schools, the children received kindness and a sound education.

I tried to reassure them that their mother and I both loved them very much, and we would always love them. Parents who denigrate each other are not uncommon in divorce, and this is most destructive and damaging to the children involved. A brilliant American divorce lawyer once said that, "nowhere are the destructive and vitriolic passions of two human beings more prevalent than in a divorce court."

Thank goodness my medical practice had me so busy that I did not have time to dwell on the past. I worked hard and played hard.

At the Valois Tennis Club where I had been a member for some years, I met Paula. She was pretty, blonde, five foot five, bright, vivacious, and an excellent tennis player. She was ten years my junior and married to an Air Canada pilot, Owen, and they had no children.

Romance was the last thing on my mind at the time. I had no intention of looking for love in any place, let alone the wrong place, but it happened. Paula had a good sense of humor, and she was fun to be with.

Since her husband was frequently out of town, Paula and I began to have lunch together. The best laid plans of mice and men often go astray! From our conversations over lunch, I gathered that Paula's husband had been involved in several affairs with flight attendants and their marriage was far from a happy one. Familiar story?

I could almost hear my patient, Stanley (the seducer of married women), whisper in my ear, "Doctor, now is your chance for seduction. Paula has the perfect profile!"

No! Absolutely not! Get thee behind me, Stanley!

But, I am ashamed to say that all of my staunch resolutions were to no avail. Paula and I wound up in bed fairly soon after meeting. She proved to be a premature ejaculator's dream come true! I seemed only to have to look at her and she would climax. Not exactly, but close! Interesting how different women are. Paula was undoubtedly the quickest responder and the sexiest woman I had ever met!

Our affair lasted almost a year, and then her husband was transferred to Vancouver, British Columbia, with Air Canada.

I had also become quite friendly with Paula's husband, Owen, who really was not a bad stick. The three of us would often go out together, and the fact that I may have been in bed with his wife just twenty minutes earlier did not seem to bother me. Perhaps there was some "Stanley" in me, a disguise with no genital conscience.

A book entitled, "The Joy of Sex, (by Alex Comfort) had just come out, and I bought a copy for Paula to read. Over the course of our one-year affair, we tried every position known to man and woman, and then some! Often we would make love in their marital bedroom, and I always insisted on turning Owen's smiling wedding photograph around!

One of Paula's favorite games was to tie me up spread eagled on their king-sized bed, and have her way with me! There was never any question as to whether Paula had climaxed or not. She was a screamer! She just kept going and going. I could not believe my luck.

Paula would often leave me tied up and inform me that her husband was due to return any moment. She obviously had a sadistic streak. One time this backfired, and Owen did arrive most unexpectedly. We heard his car in the driveway and, just in the nick of time, Paula untied me. I hurriedly dressed in their bathroom, but there was no time to return Owen's photograph to its proper position! Maybe Paula had forgotten to do that while dusting?

In the winter of 1964, my parents and I decided to take a vacation together in Jamaica. They flew from Johannesburg to Kingston, and I flew from Montréal to Kingston. We met in the customs area of the airport. My parents had their South African passports and I had my Canadian one, but they did not have a Jamaican visa.

A huge black Jamaican customs officer was just about to send them back to South Africa on the same plane when I intervened. With apartheid in full swing, most of the world regarded the racist government in South Africa as an abomination. All South Africans were tarred with the same brush.

I explained to the customs officer that my parents had sent me to Canada to pave the way for their emigration from South Africa. This was partly true, as both my father and my stepmother (dad had remarried) did soon thereafter get Canadian pink slips (the equivalent of American green cards).

Dad felt that the long-term prognosis in South Africa was poor. This seemed to placate the customs officer and he allowed them a two-week visa, but he told them that if they exceeded the time, they would immediately be put in jail.

With great relief, the three of us took off in our rented car. We checked into a bed and breakfast, run by a Mrs. Pinder, a lovely woman with a lilting Jamaican accent.

We stayed at the B&B only a few days. I learned that the Jamaican Playboy Club had recently opened, and that is where we went, pronto!

The Playboy resort was a lavish five-star, and the Jamaican bunnies were just learning to walk in high heels. Not an easy task, if you've never done it before! Within a day or two I met an attractive hotel manageress, a divorcee born in Jamaica whose name was Sylvia.

Sylvia's first marriage had not lasted long and neither did her second to a deeply religious man who had never been married before. Sylvia discovered soon into their marriage that her religious husband was a Golden and Brown shower man. They promptly divorced.

Sylvia's ex-husband's mother implored her to take him back because he supposedly had a "religious conversion" to normality. His gross sexual aberrations were now a thing of the past, she said. So, Sylvia took him back, and they remarried. Within under a month, the religious conversion evaporated and he was back to his old nasty tricks! This time the divorce was final.

Sylvia and I had a ball for the next two weeks. She knew all the locals, and we visited some of her friends who owned sugarcane farms and coconut plantations. It was interesting to see how the upper-class Jamaicans were living, pretty high on the hog!

After a week at the Playboy Club, Sylvia and I flew to Kingston, staying in a romantic hotel high up in the mountains encircling the city. We had a special suite, the "Errol Flynn" suite. At night on our front veranda, we could see the lights of Kingston town and the harbor lights twinkling in the distance.

Errol Flynn, the late actor, had spent many months in Kingston, and Jamaica was his favorite island. Errol had an eye for young ladies—very young ladies. Nevertheless, "Robin Hood" was still my hero, as he had been when I was a small boy.

My PE condition was still a handicap. Sylvia felt that a little Jamaican voodoo would cure it. She put some Pepsodent toothpaste in her mouth, mixed it with 150% proof of Jamaican rum, and performed oral sex. It stung like hell, the cure being much worse than the condition! After a few stiff Jamaican rums, we fell asleep. Next morning, with a purple looking dick, I performed marginally.

We returned to Ocho Rios, and the few remaining days were spent with my parents before they returned to South Africa.

The Jamaican Playboy Club eventually folded, as did many of the other international Playboy Clubs.

It is my sincere hope that none of my old patients will ever read this chapter! The same applies to my three brother-in-laws and their wives! I am almost too embarrassed to write it! If you were to consider me depraved and kinky, you might well be right! However, in my office with my white coat on it was all professional. It had to be. In teaching my residents, I repeatedly reinforced my advice, "Look, but never touch."

With a beautiful woman lying naked on the examining table, do not think for one moment that a lustful thought or two could not cross a doctor's mind! Ladies, you must be very naive if you think otherwise! Doctors who do not heed my advice often lose their licenses, and sometimes go to jail.

From here on, I will refer to my aggravating and distressing premature ejaculating as "my condition." This condition was with me until I was sixty-one, when a miracle happened. Towards the end of this book I will devote an addendum to this very prevalent condition, the causes, consequences, and various up-to-date modalities of treatment, both successful and unsuccessful.

The following sexual vignettes took place while I was a horny bachelor. It is my intention to devote the next few chapters to my sexual escapades. Bear with me, or I implore you to please skip this chapter altogether.

Sexual mores had changed radically in the 1960's. Smoking pot, swinging, and liberated female behavior seemed quite acceptable. AIDS only started raising its ugly head in the Western world in the early 1980's.

As a single man, many married friends would often invite me out for dinner and indulge in a certain amount of matchmaking. An extremely wealthy couple, Francois and Lorraine, invited me to go with them on their 50-foot Chris-Craft for a long weekend to the Thousand Islands.

Lorraine was a French Canadian brunette, about 5 foot four, sexy as hell, and wore low-cut blouses, mini-skirts, and swimsuits that would only be acceptable in the South of France.

Francois was a dapper Frenchman from France in his early forties, quite good looking, and accustomed to the finer things of life. Not long into our trip, I was to discover to my consternation that Francois possessed a formidable 7-inch weapon.

We had perfect weather and the scenery on the Lawrence Seaway was spectacular. The 50-foot Chris-Craft was dwarfed by the huge ships passing by. We anchored for lunch in a secluded little cove.

A pre-lunch martini or two, followed by a delicious cold lobster salad and a bottle or two of chilled French Chablis, was to set the scene for my first "menage a trois."

It occurred so naturally. After lunch the three of us were sunbathing in the nude, lying side by side on the deck, when Francois and Lorraine began to make out. Watching a couple doing what comes naturally in a beautiful setting produced some profound stirring in my nether regions! Seeing this, Lorraine came over to me. Once again, my apology of a penis let me down, so she went back to François.

I continued to see Paula, whose suspicions that her husband was having an affair were confirmed when he returned from a stopover in Vancouver. Lipstick and other incriminating evidence were found on his handkerchiefs. Confronted, he confessed, and they decided on a three-month trial separation. He went back to Vancouver and moved in with his mistress, and I saw even more of Paula.

These were blissfully happy times for me sexually, as Paula climaxed in seconds. I nicknamed her CK (Climax kid).

CK and I would often go with François and Lorraine on their Chris Craft after I had finished my office work for the day. Cocktails off Dowkers Island at sunset were a lovely way to begin summer evenings. There were many trips to the Scenery Club in lovely Montebello and return visits to the Thousand Islands. On one occasion, I offered François my credit card to gas-up the Chris Craft. In 1963, each tank took over three hundred dollars!

CK surprised me at how easily she took to swinging. Uninhibited, insatiable, and separated from her husband, she was an absolute aggressive Tigress. CK was the kind of woman men can only imagine in their wildest dreams. Adorable, she so obviously enjoyed sex with unbelievable passion!

I do believe Paula was falling in love. However, with my responsibility to my two young children and my practice, I felt that any move in that direction was premature. Once burnt, still very shy! I was never, ever going to get married again!

In February of 1964, the temperature on the West Island of Montréal was 17 degrees below zero fahrenheit. It was a crystal clear day when CK and I flew to the island of St. Barthelemy (St. Barts) for a two-week vacation. She flew on an Air Canada pass to St. Martin and, changing planes, we both continued on to St. Barts.

The approach to the airfield at St.Barts is quite treacherous, as the plane has to make an extremely rapid descent in order to land safely. As we got off our small plane, we saw several plane wrecks around the periphery of the landing strip, the result of unhappy landings! Pilots who wish to land at St. Barts need special certification, as landing requires expert precision.

The Isle de St. Barthelemy is located sixteen miles southeast of St. Martin, an easy sail if one is interested in sailing. The year-round temperatures range from 72 to 86 degrees fahrenheit, ideal for escaping Montréal's harsh winter.

St. Barthelemy is the St. Tropez of the Caribbean, a little pristine jewel. The island is French, the food every bit as good as you will find at some of the better French restaurants. There are only three policemen, and no crime had been reported for as long as anyone can remember!

We stayed at the Eden Rock Hotel on St. John's Beach, an old hotel owned by the Mayoress of St. Barts. (The Mayoress had a particularly pretty daughter who wore gayly colored pareos with nothing underneath, only briefly discernible when she nonchalantly sat down!)

There were many topless women on the beach. Some young and attractive, and some not so young and not so attractive! When entering restaurants, these topless ladies would put on appropriate attire. It was all so refreshingly natural.

We rented a small jeep and toured the island. The beaches were clean with white gleaming sands, and most were completely deserted. CK and I would go completely nude. Swimming in an ocean in one's birthday suit is an exhilarating experience.

Saline, Rockefeller, and Gouveneur were all beaches we would visit to swim and picnic. On one such occasion, CK was lying on her stomach when she felt a shadow blocking the sun. Looking up, she saw a young man with a flaccid elongated penis standing over her. She got quite a fright, as I was some distance away swimming—but all this delightful young man wanted was to borrow a cigarette lighter!

Our favorite restaurant was the L' Entrepont, close to the harbor of Gustavia. In this quaint harbor were sailboats from all over the world, and many interesting people.

Several years later, Rosemary and I visited St. Barts and it became our very favorite island in the West Indies.

Pierre and Josie were the owners and chefs of L'Entrepont, and what a fine establishment they ran. One of my favorite desserts was the frozen lemon sherbet. They would take a lemon, scoop out the inside, and fill it with sherbet, then freeze it. An ideal summer desert.

Orange pancakes baked in Gran Marnier was another delicious dessert they were famous for. This easy-to-make recipe can be found in haute cuisine recipe books. (Put them in the freezer to keep for special occasions.)

When Rosemary and I were driving through Durango, Colorado at a later time, we discovered that Pierre and Josie had left St. Barthelemy and had opened a restaurant by the same name in Durango. We dined there—a bit expensive—and it was good to see them again. They told us sadly that the reason they had left St. Barts was that some of the locals had set fire to their restaurant.

The Governor of Colorado had dined at their restaurant in St. Barthelemy many times. He was instrumental in bringing them to Colorado. What a small world!

The restaurant did not flourish as they had opened it an old reconverted church, and the "Duran-gutangs" were not very happy about that.

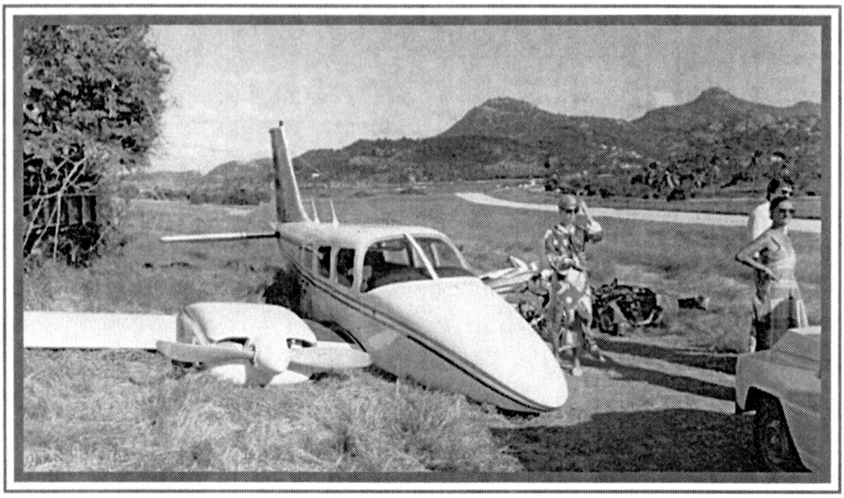

Most unhappy landing

Rosemary and I went back to our beloved little island in 2006, and what a disappointment! Spoiled, spoiled and spoiled. Hang-out for the rich, famous, nouveau riche and infamous. What a damn shame. We will never return.

Returning to my story about CK, she and her husband decided to try reconciliation, and they moved to Vancouver. (I heard by way of the grapevine that CK had later gained a lot of weight, and divorced.)

Not long after CK left, I had a series of sexual encounters. A doctor friend introduced me to a very interesting couple. John was an American and Eva a bewitching Hungarian. They lived in prestigious Upper Westmount. Both were fun people, and they had two adopted children, Stephan and Cynthia.

John and Eva were about fifteen years my senior, and photos of Eva taken in her younger days revealed an absolute knockout. They were kind, hospitable people who threw some very wild parties.

It was at one of these parties that they persuaded me to stay over for the night, as I had too much to drink. I do not remember going to bed, or very much about the rest of the evening. After I had fallen into a deep sleep, I was pleasantly awoken by Eva's warm, seductive body. It took me several seconds to remember where I was!

Eva reassured me that John did not mind, as he was a diabetic and had been impotent for many years. She quickly explained John's interesting philosophy. Rather than lose her, he thought a fair compromise was to allow her to entertain her lovers at home. I just happened to be one of the many.

They say alcohol makes one more amorous, but less effective, and this unfortunately turned out to be true. Eva told me next morning that she always preferred sex while being hung over. I hoped that her over-indulgence—she was a martini drinker—made my poor performance of the previous evening less noticeable.

The three of us had a hearty breakfast, scrambled eggs, Canadian sausage, and bacon, with slices of toast made with homemade bread. John always had a slight smile on his face and this reassured me that I was not about to die at the hands of a generous host or hardly a jealous husband!

There was a very relaxing atmosphere in the home of Eva and John, and I was a frequent visitor. Their lovely country estate was on an island in the Laurentians, not far from where Mario and Lisa had first met. The Laurentian Mountains are some of the oldest in the world, and the whole area has countless beautiful lakes. As the winter progresses and lakes freeze over, John and Eva would reach their island by automobile. In the summer, a small boat with an outboard motor was used.

Toward the end of September, the Laurentians become a mass of color. The red maples, evergreens, and various other trees with their medley of changing color bring people from all over to view the magnificent "changing of the leaves."

My dismal performance on our first night together made Eva acutely aware of my problem. But rather than give up on me as a useless tool, she set about teaching me how to make love and please a woman.

Foreplay must be gentle and prolonged. Boudoir candles, total body massage, subtle fragrant body lotions, and most importantly, accurately placed cunnilingus. The clitoris can be an elusive little devil, and often likes to play hide and seek!

Astroglide lubricant replaces saliva, and the use of the "Hatachi Magic Wand vibrator" guarantees the most anorgasmic female in the world incredible pleasure! Eva made sure she had several climaxes before allowing me anywhere near her. This took a lot of pressure off me, and helped psychologically.

She introduced me to her box of sex toys. Padded wrist and ankle restraints, cock rings, nipple clamps, and a variety of wicked looking whips! With this nasty collection, I have no doubt she could drive some of her masochistic lovers out of their minds.

Cambridge obviously never taught me any of this, and I am indebted to Eva for tutoring me in the ways of the flesh. My condition, however, remained a problem for many years to come. Now, however, I know that silent orgasms do not exist, and there is no rule that says people must have simultaneous climaxes. Ladies first, always!

Eva asked me if I would mind John watching us in their regal bedchamber. The room had a king-sized canopied bed with side, swagged curtains, and a large comfortable couch any psychiatrist would be happy to own. For a moment I hesitated, but then said, "No worries." Remember, I had a very permissive upbringing with A.S. Neil's Summerhill philosophy that virtually anything goes, including reading Shakespeare to cows!

This was a kind of consensual threesome, with a silent non-participating husband. One can rationalize anything!

Interestingly enough, when one is in the throes of sexual intercourse, one soon becomes oblivious to the presence of others. John simply relaxed on their comfortable couch, smoking his pipe, and watching his pretty wife in "delecto flagrante." The heady aroma of his pipe tobacco was the only indication of his presence.

This somewhat unusual relationship came to an end on October 16, 1965 when I met Rosemary—the special woman I was never ever going to marry!

I believe I shed my lascivious ways for good the day I met Rosemary. On October 16, 1965, I put on a new white coat and went to work in the emergency room of the Lakeshore General Hospital, which had just opened that fall.

The hospital was sorely needed as it was situated very close to TransCanada Highway where a great deal of trauma from auto accidents took place. It was the only hospital between Montréal and the Québec border with Ontario, and was a great blessing to the people of the West Island of Montréal who hitherto had to go into Montréal for medical attention and hospitalization, a distance of some twenty miles.

The emergency room was manned by family doctors such as myself who put in 24-hour shifts once or twice a month.

On October 16, 1965, I was on duty and spied an extremely attractive blonde nurse. I introduced myself. Her name was Rosemary, and I asked her to have lunch with me in the hospital cafeteria. I recall we both had chicken sandwiches!

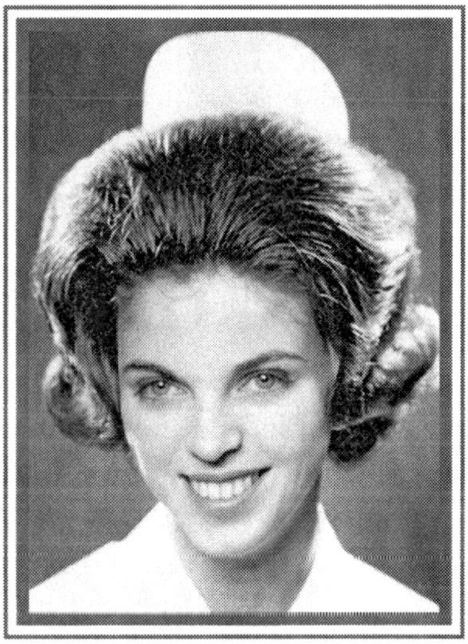

Rosemary

A "Black Velvet Party" was being held the following weekend hosted by a drug representative, and I invited Rosemary to go with me. Black Velvet is a mixture of Guinness's stout and champagne, but not understanding the meaning of the party, Rosemary wore a black velvet dress—a testimony to her endearing nature.

I spent a good deal of that evening flirting with a Playboy bunny. It was somewhat like the last dying gasps of my bachelorhood.

Rosemary was coming to the end of a torrid two-year relationship with an experienced Italian lover. Hearing this, my insecurity rose and I felt my chances with this pretty nurse were probably over before they began!

Fortified by several whiskeys, I summoned up enough courage to ask Rosemary out again. She was surprised to hear from me, having observed my lecherous behavior at the Black Velvet Party where I spent most of the evening trying to pull off the Playboy bunny's cottontail. (Did you know that those cottontails are kept in place by a press stud?)

From then on, Rosemary and I had an almost monogamous relationship. I have no intention of telling about our first sexual congress, which ended abruptly. After that most unfortunate debacle, and on her twenty-fourth birthday (December 16), Rosemary returned to her old Italian lover for a real celebration.

(In an aside, in 1991 at the age of sixty-one, I underwent surgery for prostate cancer. Shortly thereafter, my PE condition totally vanished, allowing me to become the man I had always dreamed of becoming! What a gift!)

Very early in our relationship, I made it quite clear to Rosemary that marriage was out. I was never, ever going to get married again. Little did I realize that, over the next five years, Rosemary would be my gradual undoing.

We had our first "illicit" weekend in a quaint hotel in the Laurentian Mountains at the Cuttles Tremblant Club. This rustic old pine log resort was on Lac Tremblant, a beautiful ten-mile long lake with landlocked salmon.

Never having checked in to a hotel with a woman before, I brought my ex-wife's wedding band but it was too small to fit Rosemary's finger so I threw it away! Registering was no problem and the owner, Bruce, did not seem to notice Rosemary's lack of a wedding band!

In the winter with the lake completely frozen, we walked for miles upon miles. On our return, Danny was playing in the piano bar. There was a crackling fire, comfy leather chairs, and an ugly old moose glaring down at us from its mount on the wall. We polished off a couple of single malt scotches and a glass or two of dry Chablis before going into the dining room.

We always favored a table with a long tablecloth, preferably by a picture window overlooking the frozen lake. The five-star menu featured rare roast beef and Yorkshire pudding as the Specialty of the House.

The weekend was so romantic, and over the years Rosemary and I would return often.

Too soon, I was back to seeing patients on Monday morning and doing my laundry on Monday evening. Not experienced at doing laundry, I did not realize that I was producing pink handkerchiefs, pink socks, and pink underwear. Rosemary politely pointed out that I should separate colors from non-colors! A small detail, but important!

Not long after my first date with Rosemary, I stopped having evening and Saturday morning offices. Practice had grown to the point where I felt I was not able to take on new patients. This also allowed more time with Rosemary.

The next few years, indeed the next forty-plus years, were to be some of the happiest of my life.

Rosemary and I danced to the strains of the Barry Bingham Trio at the Airport Hilton Hotel almost nightly after she came off an evening shift. In the winter, we went night skiing with nurses and doctors from the Lakeshore General Hospital. Sometimes we took Wilson and Julie to ski races at various places in the Laurentians on weekends, barely an hour away.

Living in Montréal for twenty years was a great experience, and I never thought I would leave it. Montréal and its environs had everything. Summer and winter, all had its special attractions.

We went boating on the St. Lawrence in the summer with François and Lorraine on their fifty-foot Chris Craft. There was ice sailing, cross-country, and downhill skiing in the winter. "Maple sugaring" parties (collecting maple syrup from a spout placed in the maple tree) was a great excuse for partygoers to get plastered!

Montreal had an enormous number of fabulous ethnic restaurants, all with haute cuisine—Greek, Italian, and just about every other nationality had restaurants serving delicious gourmet meals. When Rosemary and I left Montreal in 1978, there were over 700 restaurants.

In February of 1966, my mother committed suicide. She was sixty-six years old. It was totally unforeseen, and my father went into a deep depression. A marriage of thirty-six years ended tragically with a single gunshot wound to her head. I immediately flew back to South Africa.

My mother, a woman who was deathly afraid of firearms, had gone to J.F. King and Sons Gunsmith on West Street Durban, bought herself a revolver, and with one clean shot ended her life. It was ironic that my mother should choose this manner when she had enough barbiturates in her bathroom cupboard to kill half of Durban.

Mom had been seeing Adolf Simon, a German psychiatrist who had been treating her for depression for countless years. (The doctor's wife, Charlotte, worked in his front office and often wore sleeveless blouses, showing hairy armpits which, as a little boy, I thought disgusting.)

In retrospect, it was not difficult to realize that the writing had been on the wall for some time. In those days, phenobarbital was prescribed for everything, including depression. Antidepressant medication was still a long way off.

Several factors played a significant role in Mom's suicide. She had devoted most of her last ten years to taking care of her aged mother. My Granny, a simple soul who had no education, died at eighty-nine, leaving an enormous void in Mom's life.

Four years older than dad, she had let her hair go gray, which made her look even older. My mother knew dad was running around. This really broke her heart, and could have easily been the precipitating factor in her suicide. She told me once, unbeknown to dad, that she had followed him to Cape Town and had seen him with ("Elephant 8") Peter's older sister, Sonia, registering at Mount Nelson Hotel.

Sonia was recently widowed and twenty years dad's junior, a Scandinavian bombshell who could have stepped right out of a Playboy centerfold. It was just too much for the old man to resist!

Mom had so few worldly possessions—a string of pearls, pearl earrings, an inexpensive watch, a wedding ring, a small diamond engagement ring, a snap album with photos of our homes, her kids, and our dogs. That was it!

She loved gardening with a passion, and spent countless hours, when not with Granny, in our garden with her hydrangeas and other flowers. Mom introduced the white bougainvillea into South Africa.

Material things meant nothing to mother. She was much more interested in human relationships. When she lost those, she had nothing. I am finding this very difficult to write.

Anxious, kind, and gentle, mom had the common touch! Much of my own humanism and caring for people I attribute to my mother's influence. I will always miss her.

Dad and I spread her ashes in Pidgeon Valley, a wild life preserve in front of our home where she and dad had scattered Gran's ashes. The only sound to break the solitude was the mournful three-tone call of her black tragedy bird.

It took dad a long time to recover. I truly believe he loved my Mom, despite his extramarital affairs.

By the time I left South Africa, Dad was in somewhat better shape than when I arrived.

Returning to Canada, Rosemary was waiting for me at Montréal's Dorval Airport. I was thrilled to see her! She was wearing a slinky, soft wraparound skirt, with a revealing white silk blouse. Mamma Mia!

In September of 1966, Rosemary and I flew to Bermuda for a short holiday, staying at the Mermaid Beach Apartments in Southampton. These apartments were in a crescent shape facing the ocean, which magnified the sound of the waves.

It was the first holiday for Rosemary in two years, and she was exhausted. The water was warm, and the snorkeling incredible with brightly colored parrot fish and a myriad of the other colorful fish.

We rented motorcycles and toured the island from one end to the other. We loved Bermuda. Lovely British island, great restaurants, good shopping, and secluded sandy beaches. We went back many times over the years.

The friends we made in Bermuda were Bermudians. What great fun these people were! They all had boats, and we often went out to snorkel among sunken shipwrecks where ships which had met their doom off Bermuda's dangerous reefs.

Schools of barracudas watched us closely, but always kept their distance (and we ours)! They were long shiny fish with evil looking faces.

One of our Bermudian friends had a sailboat named "Climax." It was a magnificent sailboat, and we would sometimes go Spinnaker sailing. A swing seat was attached to the Spinnaker, and when the breeze came, off one would fly! Quite exhilarating and, for first-timers, quite scary. Somebody would always hold onto a rope to bring us down safely.

We were invited to several "Raft-Ups." Two or more sailboats would line up parallel to each other, and remain tied up for the night. Many of the Bermudian sailors had musical instruments, gut buckets (primitive double bass, one string), and harmonicas. Music entertained us until the wee hours of the mornings.

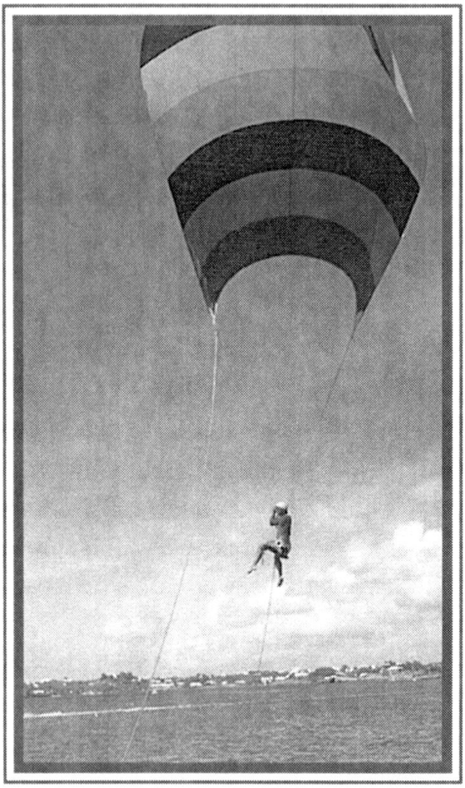

Rosemary, Spinnaker Sailing

I have never seen so much beer consumed anywhere in the world as in Bermuda, and that includes Australia, mates! The dingy in tow for empty beer cans was called snap-a-cap. Next morning, most of us woke up with hangovers. Our well-known cure, the hair of the dog, was usually a Bloody Mary or two, followed by a breakfast of fluffy Gin omelets!

On several occasions, our Bermuda friends came to visit us in Montréal during the winter. They had never seen snow!

In 1967, Montréal hosted the World's Fair, called "Expo 67." It was held in the summer and there were sixteen glorious weekends of sunshine, quite exceptional for a Montréal summer!

Rosemary and I had passports which enabled us free entry to some of the ninety pavilions of various nations. Many of the pavilions had restaurants featuring delicious ethnic food. Expo '67 was one of the most successful of the world fairs, and is still regarded fondly by Canadians, including us!

One of the magnificent features of Expo' 67 was the World Festival of Entertainment, featuring opera, ballet and theater companies alongside orchestras, jazz groups, famous Canadian pop musicians and other cultural attractions.

More than fifty million visitors attended Expo '67 at a time when little Canada's population was only twenty million, setting a record for world fair attendance which I understand still stands.

At this same time, the FLQ (Front for Liberation of Québec) terrorist organization was active, and death threats were issued to various dignitaries including American President Lyndon B. Johnson (who had attended Expo '67).

President Charles de Gaulle, master excreta disturber, created an international uproar when he shouted "Vivre le Quebec Libre" from the balcony of Montréal City Hall on July 24, 1967. That slogan to this very day is a rallying cry for the separatists in Québec who want an independent state in Canada.

1967 was referred to as the "last good year" before economic decline, and before Québec sovereignty raised a crippling economic head.

Expo '67 made us proud to be Canadians. It introduced so many people from other countries to spectacular little Canada!

In 1968, Rosemary and I bought a beautiful home on the West Island of Montréal's Lakeshore. It was three stories high—the ground floor was at lake level, the front entrance at street level with kitchen, living and dining room, and two bedrooms were upstairs. Every single room, including the bathrooms, had views of the

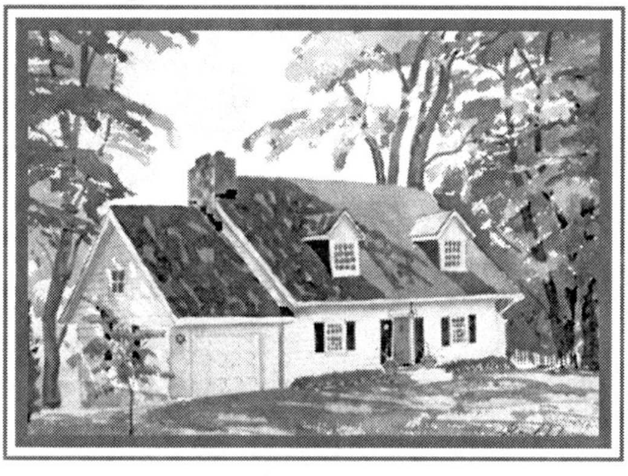

Our Lake Shore Home

lake. The front door was painted bright red and had a great big "Leo" brass doorknocker.

As winter became progressively colder, the lake froze and we often went cross country skiing for miles. Some of our friends had ice sailing boats with brightly colored sails, and we could see them skimming along the ice at high speed.

Our home had a dozen hundred-year-old trees, Elm, Maple, and Oak. We lost many of the Elm trees with Dutch Elm disease. This home was our love nest, a dream cottage!

Rosemary's parents strongly disapproved of their beautiful Catholic daughter living in sin with a divorced, dirty Protestant. (Neither Rosemary's stepmother nor her father knew of my Jewish ancestry.) And so, on February 25, 1970, Ian, who was never again going to get married, succumbed to Rosemary's irresistible charms. Why did I decide to get married again? A good question.

It is said that opposites attract, and that probably is the answer. Rosemary and I are so very different. She is bright, intelligent, very pretty, an avid reader, and a very private person. She could no more have written this kind of memoir than fly to the moon.

We grew to love each other over a four-year period, but more importantly we really liked each other. Compromise, mutual respect and caring for each other have made our last forty-two years together the ingredients for a successful marriage.

Don't kid yourself, there have been many differences of opinion over the years, usually over stupid things and my kids! Sometimes I could not even remember what it was we were arguing about.

Please do not let me give you the impression for one moment, that we have not had some wild times together. My sexy little firefly, Rosemary, can be quite a party animal on occasion. Trust me!

Although her name is frequently mentioned in many chapters of my memoirs, I have tried to respect Rosemary's privacy.

There is no one else in the world I would rather have shared these past forty-two years with than my Firefly. I hope she feels the same.

Rosemary stood by me through some difficult times with Wilson and Julie not to mention "my condition" which, fortunately, did not detract from our love. This lovely lady was a keeper, and I was not about to let her slip away!

Rosemary was twenty-eight and I was thirty-nine when we married. Rosemary's mother and father wanted to host a large elaborate wedding, but Rosemary preferred a small one with just close friends.

We decided to elope to South Africa. Dad was thrilled with the news, and wanted to make all the arrangements and pay for them. My dad loved me!

We flew to South Africa on February 23, and had an appointment to see the minister the following day. He was not exactly pleased to see us as we were not members of his Bush Baptist Church, but he did agree to marry us.

Since seasons in the Southern Hemisphere are reversed, our wedding day on February 25 was hot and humid. Rosemary had spent the previous night with Dr. and Mrs. Harry Radford in their lovely home in Kloof, a suburb of Durban. Harry had kindly offered to give Rosemary away.

The small wedding Rosemary had wanted turned out to have over two hundred guests, none of whom she knew! There were Durban celebrities, old Michaelhouse and Cape Town friends, including my buddy Dr. Jerry Steyn from University of Cape Town. Jerry was now a successful cardiologist practicing in Pretoria. Dad was my best man and, later that same year, I would be his!

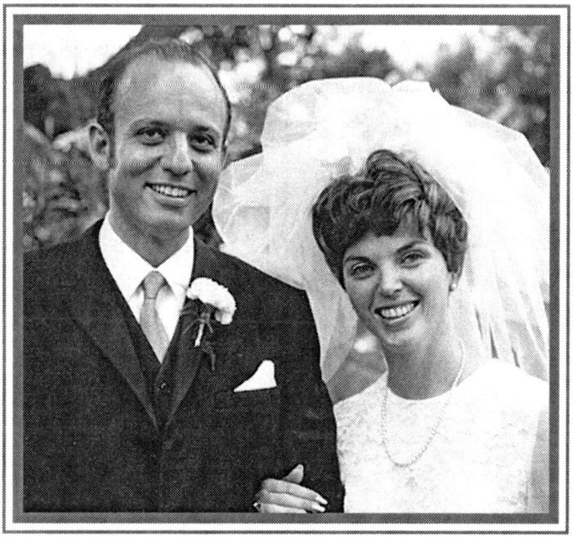

Famous Last Words!

The church service went by without a hitch and Rosemary looked stunning in her white miniskirt wedding dress. Mini-skirts had not yet reached South Africa, and her dress caused quite a stir!

Our reception was held in the prestigious Durban Country Club situated close to Durban's North Beach, surrounded by two 18-hole golf courses. Excellent wedding photos were taken in Durban's Old Fort Gardens.

Our South African guests quickly made Rosemary feel at home. Turbaned Indian waiters served a magnificent meal, accompanied by delicious dry Dom Perignon.

Cornelius, dad's cook, had brought his family down from Zululand to meet Rosemary. Cornelius had one wife and five children, and none of them had ever seen the sea. We took them down to the beach where a notice read, "For black bathers only." This was a segregated beach quite some distance away from the white beach.

The children had the time of their lives frolicking in the waters of the Indian Ocean. None of them had ever tasted ice cream, and so we all had ice cream.

Such dear people, I wonder what has happened to them in the new South Africa. One of our African American friends asked me, "Why not find out?" A very good question, but what could I say to them? I really do not know, but perhaps forlornly apologize with an agonizing question of my own. "Can you ever find it in your hearts to forgive us our sins against your parents?" I grieve for our beloved country.

One of our wedding guests, Major "Mad" Mike Hoare, was a South African mercenary employed by Tshombe (head African in the Belgian Congo at that time). Mike was born in Ireland, an accountant by profession. Tshombe paid Mike and his mercenaries in gold.

Mike once gave dad a beautiful African carved wooden chair that had belonged to Tshombe. My father was Godfather to his two boys, whom I believe are living somewhere in the United States.

Looking at the man, one would never think of Mike as a ruthless killer, but he was. He once led a group of South African mercenaries to the Seychelle Islands in an attempt at a coup, but it had a disastrous ending. Their arrival at the airport was anticipated. The mercenaries flying into the airport from South Africa were drunk and had spilled the beans. At one of the stops, a passenger had gotten off and alerted the Seychelle authorities.

The mercenaries, who were pretending to be a rugby team called "the Ancient Order of Froth Blowers," had suitcases filled with high-powered rifles, grenades, and other lethal weapons. A tremendous shootout at the airport followed, and several of Mike's comrades were killed. His brother-in-law was captured. At that moment, an Air India jet was making a landing at the Seychelles airport. Mike and the remaining mercenaries hijacked it and flew back to South Africa.

This incident placed the South African Government in a precarious position because if they had condoned this act of air piracy, no airline would ever fly into South Africa. There was some evidence that the South African Government had been backers of the failed coup, but this was never proved.

Mike and his mercenaries were jailed in Pretoria, where Mike later wrote a book. His brother-in-law was sentenced to be hanged in the Seychelle Islands, but after several grim years in jail he was set free and went back to South Africa.

Several years ago, I attempted to locate Mike in Europe, but his whereabouts were shrouded in secrecy. The mercenary old boys' club is very protective of their members, and I am sure you can understand why!

Mike had tried at one point to immigrate to Canada, but was "persona non-grata" as a result of his criminal activities.

My father had forgotten to book Rosemary and me into the Maharani Hotel and so we spent the first night of our honeymoon in his guest bedroom, next to his own room. I was reminded of my Cambridge days when the room in my new digs was next to my newlywed landlord and his wife. Only this time, it was my father listening in!

The day after our wedding, we drove up the north coast of Natal to the Hluhluwe Game Reserve, the home of the white and black rhino, for a "private honeymoon." Our accommodations were in a spotlessly clean thatch-roofed rondaval.

It was Rosemary's first visit to South Africa, and she was fascinated by the animals in Hluhluwe. The rhinos may have poor eyesight, but their hearing is acute. One should always try to keep downwind from these prehistoric beasts.

On return to Durban, I paid a brief visit to Wally Visser. In his younger days, Wally had been an outstanding rugby player for England. The "Adonis of Durban's North Beach," he had a crucial role in saving a lifeguard's life in the shark attack I had witnessed there.

Wally had been unable to attend our wedding because of his crippling Parkinson's disease. He sat alone in his darkened living room with a mask-like, expressionless face, so typical of the disease.

Wally could barely speak and when I asked him how his son Colin was, one solitary tear slowly ran down his cheek. That was his answer. Wally had never accepted the fact that Colin was homosexual. He did not want Colin ever to return to South Africa. It took a very long time for gay pride to arrive in South Africa.

Colin had a long-term significant other, but the relationship broke up after many years. I was very fond of him, my friend from Elephant 8 and best man at my first marriage in England. Colin died in Florida at age sixty-five, not having seen his father in over forty years.

Rosemary and I left lovely South Africa after a great honeymoon, and flew back to Canada. We had taken the top tier of our wedding cake to celebrate the christening of our first child (which we never had).

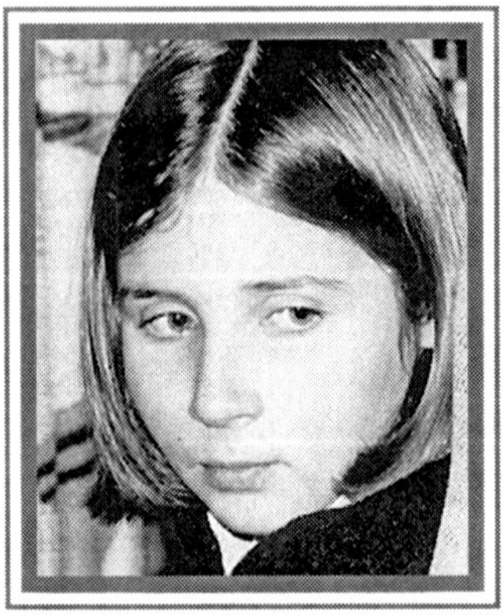

Julie!

Surprise! Julie, my daughter (then eleven), was waiting at Dorval International Airport for us. Lisa had taken Julie out of her boarding school to live with her in her new home in Westmount.

Lisa's alcoholism had reached a point where Julie did not want to live with her anymore, and so she came to live with us in our home on Old Lake Shore Road in Beaconsfield.

When I recount some of Julie's adventures, it is easy to see why Rosemary decided against having children. Neither Rosemary nor I had any idea of just how messed up Julie was.

A year or two after my mother died, dad began seeing Norah, a widow who had been a close friend of our family. They became great companions and traveled all over the world together, including visits to see us in Montréal. We really liked Norah, and our wedding in South Africa may have been the catalyst for dad's proposal to her.

Dad and Norah realized that if they had married in Durban, it would have been a colossal affair. Like Rosemary, all they wanted was a small intimate wedding.

The top tier of our wedding cake became theirs when Norah and Harry Whyte were married in the Little Church of the West in Las Vegas, Nevada on Friday, August 14, 1970. I was dad's best man and Dr. "Big" John Duffy, Professor of Anesthesiology at UCLA, gave Norah away. They held a champagne and caviar reception at Caesar's Palace with just a few close friends. It was good to see these two special people so happy and in love.

After all those years, I was still unable to read. In 1971 at the age of forty-one, I took a speed-reading course hosted by Evelyn Wood in the Embassy Hotel on Sherbrooke Street, Montréal.

At the time, I was barely reading one hundred words a minute with no recall, but within the first three-hour session I read five hundred words a minute and could tell you exactly what I just read! While most of the class did considerably better than this, they were not dyslexic.

The strategy was simple. Just use the tip of the right index finger as a pacer, going from left to right below each line! One's eyes followed the "finger pacer."

You have no idea how much being able to read meant to me. My heartfelt thanks to Ms. Evelyn Wood.

The Front de Liberation du Quebec (Quebec Liberation Front) was a left wing terrorist group in Canada responsible for more than two hundred bombings and the deaths of at least five people. This very serious situation came to a head on October 5, 1970 when the FLQ kidnapped James Richard Cross, the British Trade Commissioner.

Five days later, the Minister of Labor and Vice Premier of Québec, Pierre Laporte, was kidnapped and later murdered. Prime Minister Pierre Elliott Trudeau instituted the "War Measures Act." That act was the first and only time a province had used this legislation in peacetime.

As things transpired, the FLQ movement involved considerably fewer people than had hitherto been suspected. Nevertheless, it was an anxious time for Canada and a great relief when the ringleaders were rounded up and either jailed or allowed to go to Cuba.

While all this was going on, I was practicing family medicine on the Lakeshore in what amounted to an English ghetto. My French patients all spoke English and, as a result, my French was nonexistent.

What concerned me greatly was what was happening to my children. I was trying to play both mummy and daddy, with Rosemary's help, but any attempt to discipline Julie resulted in her running off to see her mummy.

Mummy Lisa, meanwhile, was inebriated much of the time and had not the remotest idea of what Julie was up to!

We had once discovered to our horror, for example, that Julie and her girlfriend had gone into a room at the Embassy Suites with two strangers they picked up at some bar.

Both Julie and her friend looked considerably older than they were. Their pick-ups had plied them with alcohol and pills (date rape drugs). While I never got the full story, apparently the two girls spent the night with these men. They were lucky to come out alive.

The episode created a difficult situation in our home and, for better or worse, at age thirteen I put Julie on the birth control pill as I did not want an already complicated situation to get further complicated.

Julie lived with us for about three years, but it was just not working out. Rosemary's attempts to keep our home spick and span were frustrated on every turn. Julie's room was always a mess, with wet towels on the bed and heaven alone knows what else! Sound familiar? On the other hand, I was in the middle, trying to play mummy and daddy in a futile attempt to compensate for Julie's messed up childhood.

Lisa denigrated both Rosemary and me. She blamed Rosemary for our marriage breakup when I only met Rosemary well after our divorce. It is no wonder second marriages often end in divorce.

When Julie was sixteen, I set her up in an apartment below my office. This way, I could see her every day and I was just a phone call away at night.

This seemed a reasonable solution, under the circumstances. It was also a golden opportunity for Julie to grow marijuana between tomato plants in the backyard of my office! Marijuana grows very well in Québec, and the Québec provincial police were constantly closing down farms and arresting people.

Eventually, Julie went back to Carlton University, leaving behind a dozen healthy six-foot marijuana plants.

If you have children or grandchildren, eventually illegal drugs may well enter their lives in one way or another. It is not my intention to go into the hotly debated question as to whether marijuana should be legalized, but here are a few of my own observations.

Marijuana has a wide spectrum of action, and may have some medical benefit. It may possibly help people with multiple sclerosis, nausea associated with chemotherapy, and pain from terminal malignancies. However, it remains in the system for a month or longer and can create problems for recreational users who mix pot and booze. The additive effect of booze and marijuana slows reaction time and can seriously impair cognition, resulting in an increased number of traffic accident fatalities.

Apart from increased appetite (the munchies), there is the "amotivational syndrome." An insidious mental lethargy occurs which, in a highly competitive world, is of no help. Many regular recreational users of pot appear to be oblivious of this side effect, and never reach their full potential in life.

The brain, our computer, is a delicate and fragile organ. It can be thrown out of kilter and sometimes damaged irreparably. Marijuana is just one of a whole slew of substances that can result in possible brain damage.

On this subject, one of my woman patients asked me to examine her significant other. He was a well-dressed, forty-two year old executive, complaining of headaches and memory loss. He denied any drug use and his physical examination did not reveal much, so I ordered a CT scan of his brain.

An hour or so later, the radiologist phoned me asking for the patient's age. When I told him he was forty-two years old, he was astonished. The man's brain was less than half the size of a normal brain for that age. To cut a long story short, he had been snorting cocaine for several years, and this was his legacy. His brain function was permanently damaged, and his memory history.

People never think these kinds of things can ever happen to them, but they can and do.

My son, Wilson, was living at a boarding school in Ottawa. During Wilson's last year in high school at age seventeen, he began hearing voices and felt people were following him. I took him to see several psychiatrists, but none of them realized that the poor fellow was developing schizophrenia.

Ottawa was 106 miles from Montréal and I regularly drove there after a long day in the office to comfort Wilson, returning home on a dangerous three-lane highway at night.

Wilson had paranoid schizophrenia. He had a complete schizophrenic breakdown in July of 1978 while on a summer job in James Bay where he worked at a massive hydroelectric plant in northern Québec. His behavior became bizarre and he was convinced the people he was working with were planning to kill him. It did not take the supervisor long to realize that Wilson was in deep trouble mentally.

Wilson was taken to the Montréal General Hospital and admitted to the psychiatric unit where he remained for the next three months. During that time, he was given electro-convulsive therapy (shock treatment), as his diagnosis was still uncertain.

After his discharge, Wilson returned to the University of London Ontario, and managed somehow to obtain a BA. He then applied to St. Thomas' Medical School in London, and flew over for an interview. This time the old boy grapevine was unable to help, as he just did not have the marks. A student from Bermuda took the last remaining opening and, in retrospect, this was a blessing.

When I was still at Cambridge, one of my fellow medical students had a schizophrenic breakdown. I knew the chap. He had been at Michaelhouse with me, a big fellow who received a heavyweight boxing blue at Cambridge. In the anatomy lab, I had spent much time trying to help him but he was never able to continue with his studies.

Schizophrenia is a devastating disease, and only one who has had a close encounter with a schizophrenic can possibly know how hard it is to live with this disease. Schizophrenics are on a very different wavelength, often refusing their medication and winding up yet again in hospital.

Wilson eventually became litigious, suing not only his own psychiatrist in London Ontario but me for lack of financial support! Somehow, he managed to persuade an attorney to take on his ridiculous, defenseless cases.

Now fifty-two, Wilson has never been able to hold down any kind of meaningful job. He lives in a one-bedroom apartment on the third floor of a government-subsidized apartment building in London, Ontario. The apartment is as drab and barren as his life—no colorful pictures on walls, and no semblance of warmth.

The Canadian government provides a modest disability income, and free medical and dental care. His current girlfriend is a drug addict who lost custody of her child. This young woman told Wilson she would move in with him, but needed $3000 for the move. Somehow he had managed to squirrel away this nest egg and give it to her, but she never moved in!

The girlfriend periodically hits Wilson up for more money because she "needs morphine for a cancer she has developed." The situation is very chaotic and a complete tragedy.

Paranoid schizophrenia is probably the most potentially dangerous form of the disease. Victims are incapable of forming any type of long lasting friendship because of their paranoia. They are convinced that people are "out to get 'em," which may or may not be true!

Such sick people are totally out of touch with reality, and often hear voices instructing them to kill. Such realities defy rational thinking, and therein lies the problem. The paranoid schizophrenic is quite capable of killing and they often do. Sometimes there are warning signs and sometimes not. Law enforcement is usually in a quandary as how to handle these disturbed people. Unless there is imminent danger to themselves or other people, law enforcement is unable to intervene until it is too late.

A recent news report concerned thirty-two people killed by a deranged gunman at Virginia Tech, the largest campus shooting in American history. The gunman had grudges against rich people, and yet he was able to go out and buy two revolvers at five hundred dollars each.

The gunman could have easily been a paranoid schizophrenic, but up to that point in time had apparently no history of violence. People often look for explanations where there are none.

Often schizophrenics become alienated from their families. With the advent of newer antipsychotic drugs, a new set of problems may appear—the inability of the "cured" schizophrenic to re-enter the family circle after years of antisocial behavior. Their families have moved on, and these unfortunates may no longer be welcome.

My heart breaks whenever I see Wilson. I have stopped giving him money because it goes directly to his drug-addicted girlfriend who refuses rehabilitation. Speaking to Wilson's psychiatrists on several occasions, it became obvious that he was never a candidate for any of the newer antipsychotic drugs because of his lack of compliance with follow-up blood tests.

In 1976, Montréal was host to the Summer Olympics. The weather was fabulous, and Rosemary and I had front-row seats for the opening and closing ceremonies which were spectacular. Seeing all those young smiling and waving athletes from all over the world coming to compete in Montréal was inspirational.

Rosemary sat ringside when Nadia Comaneci, the fourteen year-old Rumanian, scored seven perfect tens and won three gold medals. Cuba's Alberto Juantorena was the first man to win both the 400m and 800m. In the 800m, he was so far ahead of the others that, as he kept looking back over his shoulder, there was no one even close!

Regrettably, the Olympic Stadium remains a lasting monument to the huge deficit created by the 1976 Summer Olympics. The retractable roof had never worked, and the whole shooting match almost bankrupted the City of Montréal.

In the fall of 1976, the Liberal Government of Québec was defeated by Québec's first Separatist Government.

It was a Monday, and Rosemary and I were at a diplomatic cocktail party hosted by the Consul of Guatemala when the news came over television that the Québec Separatist Government had won the election. Many consuls, including the United States, were attending the party—which came to a grinding halt at the news. The guests were visibly shaken, some even crying. In retrospect, these people knew what was in store for Québec.

By summer of 1977, the Parti Quebecois Government under the leadership of Rene Levesque passed Bill 101. "The Charter of the French Language" came into being, the details of which often defied rational explanation.

Foremost, the language in Québec was French and English was barely tolerated. French signs had to be larger than English signs, and placed above them. The French-speaking police (tongue troopers) checked on this sort of thing, and reported infractions to the authorities. Anyone not complying was fined, and sometimes put out of business.

Captions on Québec license plates still say, "Je me souvien"—translated, "I remember" (all the years of English injustice, implied).

Doctors wishing to practice in the Province of Québec had to have a certificate demonstrating their proficiency in the French language, which included medical French. In my case, my Québec license went back to 1961, and I was "grandfathered" in.

The English residents of Québec began to realize that they were in the minority and began to feel like second-class citizens. On the West Island where I practiced, panic set in and people were selling their homes for a fraction of the true value.

All sorts of restrictions were also enacted pertaining to schooling, and I did not have the first idea of how this complicated formula worked—for example, who was allowed to go to which schools!

There were some other very important financial reasons why Rosemary and I decided to leave Québec. A family doctor could only make so much money. Every three months, a financial ceiling was placed on our gross income, and if this amount was exceeded we would be taxed at ninety percent! An impossible situation. The amount of money we received was a gross figure, out which one had to pay all running expenses—wages for secretary, nurse, and everything else, which came to fifty percent of the gross. With the Canadian taxation system, we were left with precious little money.

Many of the larger companies and banks transferred their head offices to Toronto. Québec doctors such as myself began to move to the United States or other parts of Canada. The vibrant city of Montréal had suffered a serious setback.

Restaurants closed and many shops went out of business. To walk down Crescent Street, previously a street with so much charm and activity, and to see so many shops and restaurants empty, was a very depressing sight.

Rosemary and I saw the writing on the wall and during a holiday to Durban in the fall of 1977, we sat down with dad and discussed our possible future plans.

Dad had been to Arizona on several occasions, and always visited his old friend, Senator Barry Goldwater. I wrote a letter to Senator

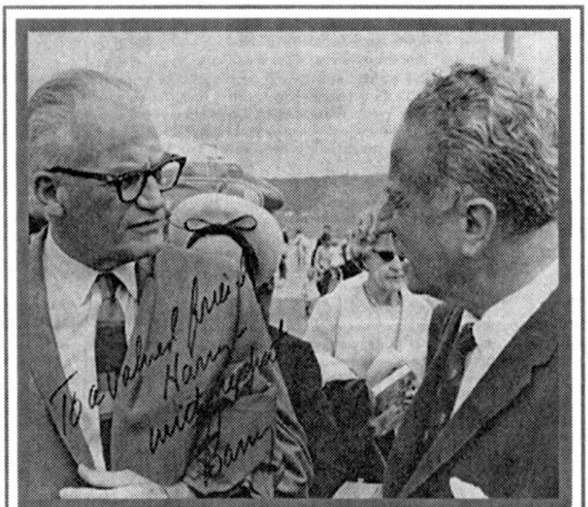

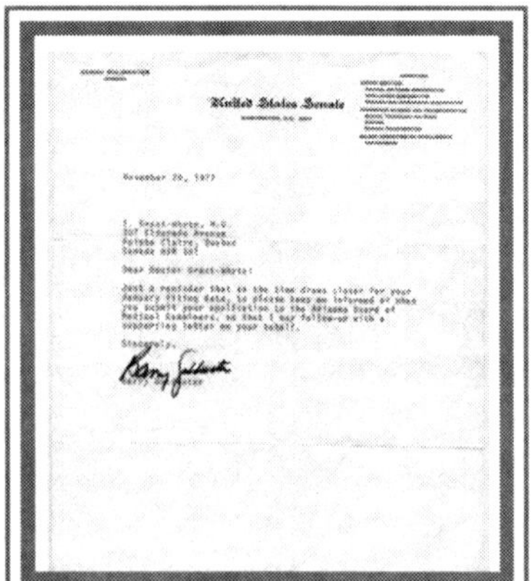
United States Senate

[illegible]

Dear Doctor [illegible]:

[illegible]

Sincerely,

Barry Goldwater

Barry Goldwater and Dad . . . and the Goldwater letter

Goldwater, and my father signed it. The letter was helpful in obtaining an interview with the Arizona Board of Medical Examiners.

Since the Board required me to pass an oral examination, Rosemary and I flew to Phoenix in January of 1978. We thought we had died and gone to heaven! What a climate change from the cruel Québec Winter! The silhouettes at night of Camelback and Mummy Mountains resembled cardboard cuttings set against the backdrop of a star-studded sky. Never had we ever seen so many shooting stars!

After a successful oral examination (Arizona license 10311), Rosemary and I set off to explore the magnificent State of Arizona.

We rented a car and set out into the vast Arizona desert with its surrounding mountains and enormous Saguaro cacti looking almost human, their arms pointing toward the cloudless sky. It is said that if the arms point downward, the unfaithful spouses of the indian wives were buried beneath. If the Saguaro arms point upward—as most do—it has the appearance of giving "the finger" to the relentlessly hot desert sun.

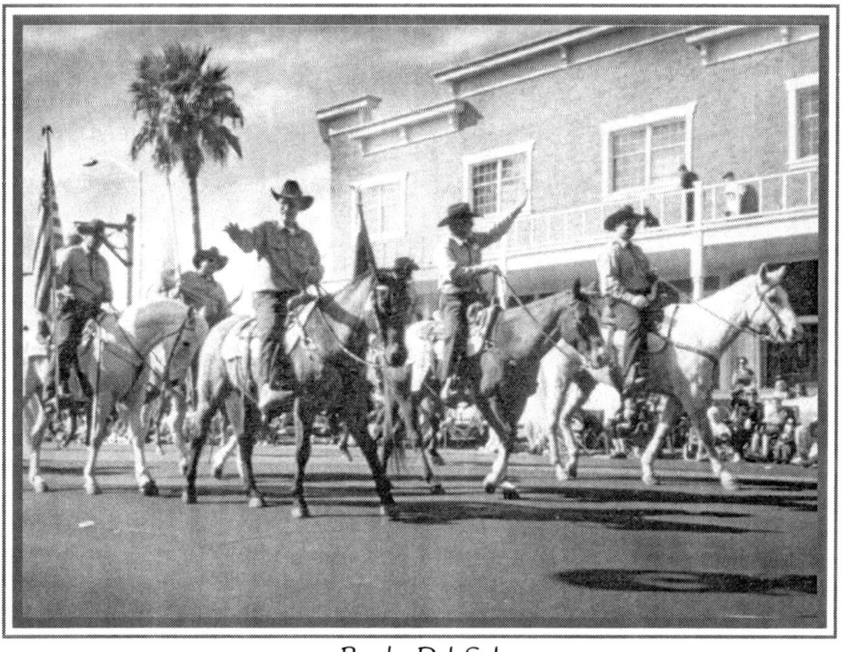

Prada Del Sol

This is cowboy country, no doubt about it. At every turn, sites had whimsical names such as Bloody Basin or Dead Man's Wash. The 12,000-foot snow-covered San Francisco Peaks dominate the horizon, and the eerily enchanting Red Rocks of Sedona with their incredible rock formations are breathtaking. Sedona is only a two-hour drive from Phoenix, and an absolute must for Arizona visitors.

We drove further North to visit one of the Seven Wonders of the World, the Grand Canyon. This enormous chasm defies description and is billions of years old. Here, one feels very insignificant in the scheme of things.

We were so enthralled by Sedona that we decided to spend three wonderful days in this breathtakingly beautiful little tourist town. Red rocky buttes (small mountains) surround the tiny town with its art galleries and restaurants. The area is believed to be spiritual, a haven for "New Agers" who believe that a mystical vortex beckons.

Mexican food was a new experience for us, and we enjoyed a Mexican restaurant named Oaxaca, washing down quesadillas and chimichangas with salty margaritas.

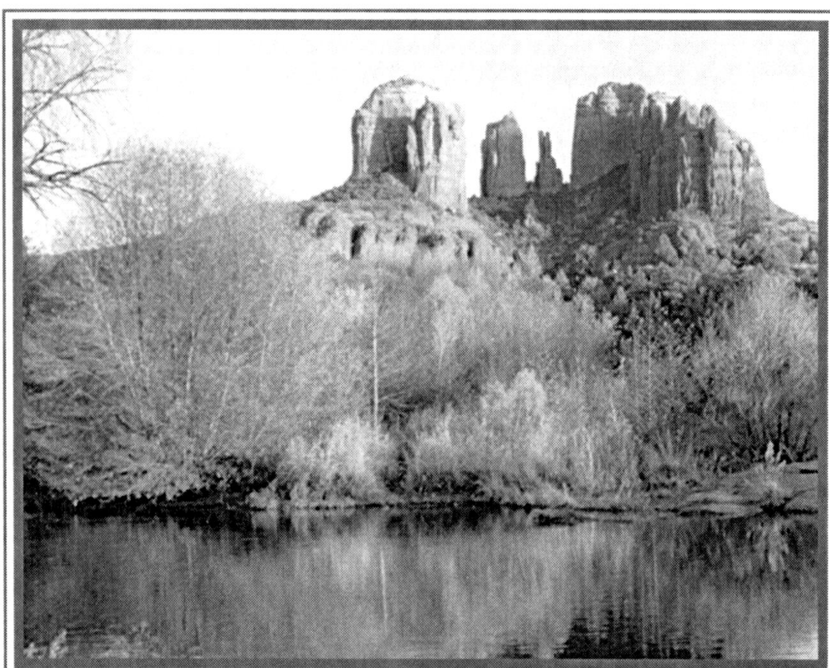

Sedona, Arizona

We drove on to the ghost town of Jerome, an old mining town converting to an artist colony. Jerome sits atop a mountain with wonderful views of the desert below stretching as far as the eye can see. The "House of Joy" was once an old whorehouse frequented by the miners of yesteryear, and now converted into a wonderful restaurant.

Tucson is a few hours' drive from Phoenix and a much smaller city than Phoenix. With quite a bit of desert landscaping, Tucson had a somewhat scrubby appearance at that time, but has since begun to develop and grow nicely.

Rosemary and I prefer big city life with theaters, good restaurants, and all the trappings that go with it, and Phoenix has it all! Fabulous Phoenix—now the fifth largest city and the fastest growing state in the United States. Old-time Arizonans grumble at this fact, but fact it is.

After our three-week visit in Arizona, there was no doubt in our minds. Arizona was the place for us!

We returned to Montréal and began to make our plans for relocation to Arizona. We obtained green cards and rented our beautiful home on the lake to friends for two years. My practice was turned temporarily over to a first-class physician, also for two years. In other words, if things do not work out for us in the United States, we could return to our home and practice in Montreal. We had not burned our bridges.

Julie's boyfriends left much to be desired. One such boyfriend whom she seemed particularly smitten with was Pierre LeDUC. Pierre was once apprehended at Heathrow Airport with a suitcase full of drugs, and jailed. His family was not wealthy, and they had to mortgage their home to provide bail for their son.

Julie flew to England with the bail money and they left together—skipping bail. But this was nothing compared to what she got up to next.

Shortly before Rosemary and I left for Arizona, Julie came to talk with me. She and her current boyfriend were going to holiday in Columbia for a few weeks. This greatly surprised me, as it seemed an unlikely place for a vacation. (I warned her that I would not be able to get her out of a Colombian jail.) Regardless of my suspicions, she reassured me that everything was on the up and up. A month later, Julie returned to Canada with this story:

The purpose of the so-called holiday was to teach a new technique for processing hashish to a Colombian general and his henchmen. In the group were two Australians, two Brits, Julie, and her boy friend, Richard. Their hideout was in a remote mountainous part of Columbia, and in order to reach their destination the group had to travel through jungle on dirt roads.

One night, Julie overhead a conversation between the Brits and the Australians saying that they were going to kill Richard, and what they intended to do with Julie you can well imagine.

Julie and Richard were not about to sit around and wait for this to happen! In the middle of the night, they managed to steal five thousand dollars of the general's money, and make a silent getaway. Realizing their escape time was limited and the airports would all be closely watched, they went to a Colombian resort town, Barranquilla, and put up in the five-star El Prado Hotel.

After partying for a week on the general's money, they returned to Canada by a circuitous route, avoiding airports. One can only imagine what could await a beautiful young blonde girl in one of those Colombian hellholes.

The other part of this story involves Richard's parents, a British couple who lived in Amsterdam and owned an antique store. They decided to set sail for Australia in their fifty-foot sailboat. Richard's parents were not heard from again, and were presumed lost at sea.

Several million dollars of life insurance would go to the children in the event of the couple's death. Seven years after the parent's disappearance, they were declared dead. The life insurance company was obliged to pay up.

Miraculously, the parents suddenly appeared in Australia shortly after the life insurance company had paid the children!

Richard began to live pretty high on the hog, racing "Formula One" cars and making frequent trips to and from Johannesburg where he was involved in illicit diamond buying.

Julie recently told me that Richard had been murdered. Might we call his a short, but not so sweet life?

Arizona

- 1978 -

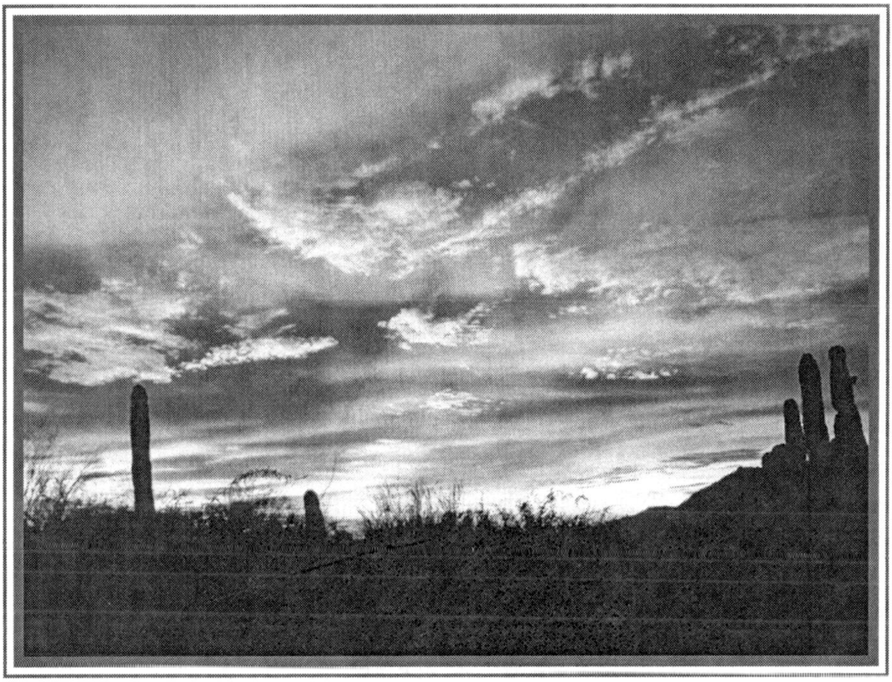

Many a flower is born to blush unseen,
and waste its fragrance on the desert air.

Farewell, Montreal! At the age of forty-eight, leaving Canada was a big step for me. I had a booming practice, a beautiful home on the lake, and many wonderful friends. There were several farewell parties. But despite our misgivings at a major change and unknown future, we looked forward to the move.

It was stinking hot when we arrived in Phoenix in July of 1978. The temperature was 115 degrees fahrenheit, and we had never experienced anything quite like it—much like stepping from the plane into an oven.

But there we were—with eleven suitcases and Dougall, our dog. Dougall missed his connecting flight in Chicago, but made it on the next one—none the worse for wear.

We had temporary reservations at Camelback Country Club and Spa. The hotel has a beautiful view of the famous Camelback Mountain, which looks amazingly like a Camel's humped back. The head has an outcrop of rock resembling a praying monk. Thus the name, Praying Monk.

Before leaving Montréal, I had arranged to take over Dr. Tommy Brown's medical practice in Phoenix. Tom was a surgeon moving on to specialize in anesthesiology at the University of Arizona in Tucson.

We rented his large office situated close to Central Avenue in Phoenix (a difficult location for patients to find!). I had signed a rental lease for five years and, in retrospect, it was not my smartest decision.

We also signed a lease agreement at the Regency House Apartments, a high-rise building near my office with lovely quarters on the nineteenth floor. It was a furnished two-bedroom apartment with maid service and great views of South Mountain. From our back balcony, we could also see Camelback Mountain.

Dougall soon adjusted to the elevator at Regency House. He enjoyed his jaunts to the ground floor where the dogs had their special place called "K9 Corral" to do business, complete with a bright red fire hydrant.

Outside, the large swimming pool was seldom used by anyone but me, and I have continued to swim 2000 meters daily for the last thirty-plus years.

The practice I took over from Tom turned out to be a disappointment, almost nonexistent, with only a few remaining patients. This scenario essentially meant that I was starting a practice from scratch—no easy matter in an area inundated with doctors where even specialists were doing general practice. It was a dog-eat-dog type of situation, so to speak!

The only referrals I received from doctors were drug addicts, and the stories the druggies came up with to get amphetamines and other narcotics were often "creative" indeed. I was apparently the new sucker doctor in the area (and their checkbooks were often conveniently left in the car)!

One such druggie came in with "excruciating pain," carrying his own gallbladder x-rays revealing multiple gallstones. He was from another state and desperately needed a morphine injection, he said, to tide him over until he could get back to his regular doctor. Yes, of course.

Rosemary worked in our office as both nurse and front desk receptionist. She soon got wise to the stories and instructed the telephone callers upfront that I will not prescribe amphetamines or narcotics. This kept only a few away.

The telephone hardly ever rang. When it did, it was often a wrong number. Having left a magnificent practice in Montréal where I had not accepted new patients in ten years, our new situation was depressing.

In the first six months of our practice in Phoenix, I grossed $20,000 (with expenses of $30,000). This unhealthy financial situation caused me to lose a lot of weight and develop a pronounced tremor in my hands. I wondered if stress was causing me to drink too much, and decided to run a series of blood tests on myself. Diagnosis: Overactive thyroid.

The treatment for hyperthyroidism was radioactive iodine which knocks out the thyroid gland completely, making it necessary to take supplemental thyroid for life.

Things went from bad to worse. I visited various nearby pharmacies, handing out my business cards to pharmacists, asking them to refer patients who were looking for a family doctor.

In time, Rosemary and I became somewhat settled and found a measure of enjoyment in our new country. Arizona is a state to fall in love with and we did. The nearby Camelback Mountain is a popular spot for hikers and from the top one has spectacular panoramic views of the city and, over the years, we would often climb this mountain.

We bought a little book called "The Best Hundred Restaurants in Phoenix," and each Saturday evening we visited one of these restaurants for a treat. But it was overall a difficult start for us, and the practice continued to remain stagnant. We were almost broke.

A life insurance company situated fairly close to my office sent me a few clients for life insurance examinations. One day, an agent from that company, Clyde Macdonald, telephoned me to say his father had died unexpectedly. His father, Dr. Lloyd Macdonald, was a well-known Phoenix physician who had practiced medicine for thirty-five years in Phoenix.

Mr. Macdonald asked me, "Would I like to buy his practice?" Thanking him, I told him I was in the process of going bankrupt and regretfully was not able to help. Fifteen minutes later, he telephoned me back and said, "The practice is yours for free, if you want it." This was the first of several very lucky breaks!

He asked if I would employ his late father's nurse, Terry, for three months to help with the transition of his dad's patients to my practice. Terry had worked for Dr. Macdonald as his nurse for 35 years, and was an absolute gem. She often blew my trumpet to all my newly acquired patients.

When Terry left after three months, I gave her a beautiful gold bracelet from South Africa, a memento I had inscribed, "Terry 1943-1978. Sincere thanks, Lloyd Macdonald." Terry, her husband Larry, and their children and grandchildren, all became my patients.

A second lucky break followed when a Dr. Marlowe had a severe stroke and was pleased to have me take over her practice. Dr. Marlowe's nurse of many years had been a friend of Terry's.

Not long after taking over our practice, we had a break-in at the office. Prescription pads and an expensive microscope were stolen. It was the possible work of a drug addict who wanted to forge prescriptions for narcotics. We boarded up the area of his break-in and, believe it or not, the bugger returned the next night to steal more!

Now in need of a microscope, I noticed an ad in The Round-Up, a monthly medical journal, concerning a Bausch & Lomb microscope for fifty dollars. I telephoned, and said that I would buy the microscope sight unseen! The doctor's wife on the other end of the line suggested I should look at it first.

The next morning I drove to their home to view the microscope. Dr. Alan Magid met me at the door. He was a retired family doctor, bald as a billiard ball! He sat me down in his study and hauled out a dusty box containing a magnificent microscope.

"What sort of doctor are you?," he asked.

"Family doctor, the same as you."

"What do you charge for an office visit?"

"$25.00."

He said gruffly, "That's far too much. I only charged $15.00."

"Dr. Magid," I said, "I did not pull this figure out of thin air! I take the highest and the lowest in the area, and go in the middle. That's where the $25.00 comes from."

He thought for a moment, somewhat placated, and then said, "Fair enough. What do you think are in all those boxes on the floor around the room?"

"I have a feeling they may be patients' charts, Dr. Magid."

"You are quite right. Would you like to have them?"

Would I like to have them!? In one visit, and fifty dollars for a microscope, I had suddenly inherited five hundred families! It was another wonderful lucky break for us.

Dr. Magid asked me to write a letter, which he signed, and Rosemary later sent the letters off to the five hundred families.

"It is with great sadness, after fifty years in practice, that I have decided to retire. Doctor Ian Whyte, a Cambridge University graduate and a kind and competent doctor, will be taking over my practice. Sincerely, Alan Magid, MD."

Dr. Magid and his wife later became patients of mine.

It was just before Christmas of 1978 when Doctor Rodger Davis came to my office. Dr. Davis had been in practice for over forty years in the Phoenix area and wished to retire.

Dr. Davis began his practice in 1938 when Phoenix was just a small dusty cowpoke town in the desert. He wore cowboy boots and immediately put his feet up onto my desk, complaining that his varicose veins were killing him.

He laid six charts on my desk and said, "Ian, you have to take the bad with the good." The charts belonged to some of his elderly addicted patients, some in their eighties, who for years had been taking large amounts of barbiturates and opiates prescribed by Dr. Davis and other doctors.

(Dr. Davis was also a bush pilot and an FAA examiner. He arranged for me to become an FAA examiner, even though I was not a pilot.)

His wife, Dorothy, had been diagnosed with lung cancer, and Dr. Davis asked me if I would look after her. I made many house calls to their hundred-acre farm in Carefree, some twenty miles north of Phoenix. Their farm was located in a beautiful hilly terrain with awesome rock formations.

Lung cancer is a relentless disease, and as Dorothy's condition worsened I alleviated her pain with a medication called the Brompton Cocktail. The ingredients of this old pain medication were formulated in the Royal Brompton Hospital in London, primarily a chest hospital. The elixir was a pleasant cherry flavored concoction of morphine or heroin, cocaine and ethyl alcohol. It was used to stop pain from resurfacing, and was to be taken on a regular basis.

Dorothy passed away in her home with little pain under six months from her initial diagnosis. Her husband went into a tremendous depression and later regrettably took his own life.

It concerned me having to prescribe large amounts of narcotics to the elderly patients I had inherited. I wrote a letter to the Arizona Board of Medical Examiners, explaining the situation and asking them for their advice. Their response was quick, informing me that I should go on prescribing the same amount as previous doctors had prescribed!

My office was far bigger than I needed and Clyde McDonald, an Omega insurance agent, referred a young man by the name of John Temple to me. John needed office space.

John was an ex-Vietnam veteran, well built, and women could not resist him! He had been a paramedic in Vietnam and had hired some very good-looking young women to do insurance examinations for life insurance companies.

The young women would go to homes and offices, fill out questionnaires, check blood pressure, pulse, height, weight and urine analyses on clients who were taking out life insurance for under $500,000. Insurance over this amount required an examination from an MD, such as me.

John was a charmer, and we immediately hit it off. I rented half of my office space to him, which took a big bite out of the rent. But just as important was the presence of John's young women insurance examiners. Their peels of laughter as they came and went created a happy and lively workplace that Rosemary and I both loved.

When I first came to Arizona to take my Arizona license oral examination, I had made a note of my examiners' names, or so I thought! I had been on call at all times with my beeper, and wanted to join my examiners for weeknight and weekend coverage in a group practice.

The initials of one of my examiners were "J.L." and I knew that the surname began with a "G," so I looked in the Maricopa County Medical Society directory and found a doctor with the matching initials, "J. L. Grubbe." This had to be one of the examiners I was looking for!

I went to Dr. "J.L. Grubbe's" office one afternoon with my curriculum vitae, and sat down in his waiting room. But when Dr. Grubbe came out, I realized that he was not one of my examiners. He was a pleasant older physician who took my curriculum vitae with a somewhat puzzled expression, and I suppose he wondered what the hell I was doing there. I wondered the same thing, feeling like a complete idiot!

To my great surprise, two weeks later Dr. Grubbe phoned, asking me to meet him in the doctor's lounge of Phoenix Baptist Hospital. The hospital had just started a three-year residency program for family doctors. Dr. Grubbe was the head of the department, and he asked if I would consider teaching residents a few mornings each week.

I had never taught before, and I asked Dr. Grubbe if I could accompany him on his rounds to watch him teach in the family practice unit.

After one hour of observing him, I knew I could teach. I accepted the offer.

This was another new experience for me, and for the next ten years I taught the doctors of tomorrow the art of medicine which I had learned at Cambridge.

By the end of one year in Arizona, Rosemary and I felt that good fortune had certainly been ours—four well-established practices, a teaching post, someone to pay half the office rent, and pretty girls to look at all day long!

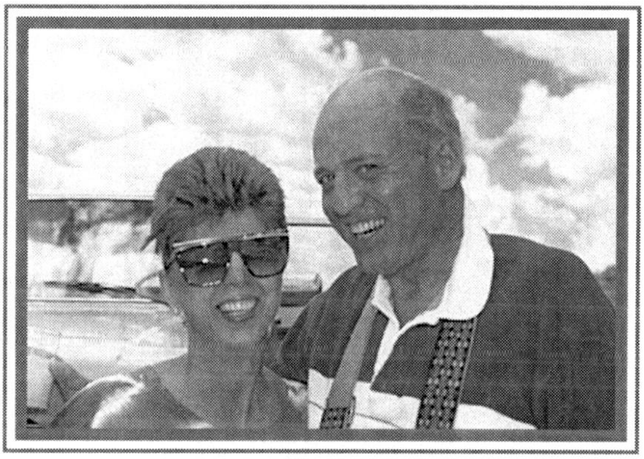

Life has been good to us!

There was no doubt that Arizona was the place for us, so Rosemary returned to Montréal to fetch our furniture and sell our home. We then moved into a larger, three-bedroom apartment on the twelfth floor of our Phoenix high-rise, with the same lovely views.

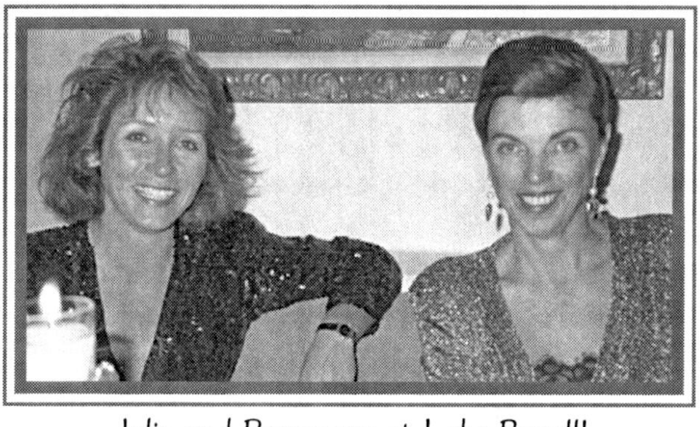

Julie and Rosemary at Lake Powell!

In need of a well-earned holiday, we decided to spend a week with John Temple, his wife Joyce, and three other couples on beautiful Lake Powell. Julie flew down from Montréal to join us on our first house boating experience. Lake Powell is a man-made lake situated on the Utah/Arizona border, approximately 180 miles long with many canyons going off in various directions.

House boating is popular in the summer and Lake Powell is breathtakingly beautiful. Personally, I feel it is every bit as impressive as the Grand Canyon.

John brought his speedboat for waterskiing and fishing. We all chipped in to buy food, countless cases of beer, and enough hard liquor to last a year. The weather was perfect when we arrived at the little town of Wahweep and picked up our houseboat at the marina. Off we sailed!

We anchored for the night in a private cove. The houseboat was well equipped with stove, fridge, and a barbecue on deck. Most of us slept up top on the houseboat, as it was cooler there. The pitch-black night on the lake was brilliantly lit with stars, and lying on deck I felt I could almost touch them.

Dawn comes early, and we began our days with Bloody Marys. Boating and drinking have (not wisely) always gone together, and house boating was no exception.

My daughter, Julie, was a drop-dead gorgeous young woman, and this was not lost on John's wife, Joyce. She was none too pleased when John took Julie in his speedboat after breakfast for a day of fishing. Fish, however, did not feature on that night's menu.

Shortly after we had gone to bed that night, the silence was shattered by John's terrified scream coming from the cabin below—"Ian! Ian! Help!"

Stumbling down the stairs, I ran into the cabin and saw John's enormous body pinning down Joyce—who held an eight-inch metal ice pick in her hand! There was no doubt Joyce (who was stone sober) had every intention of killing him but, in the nick of time, he managed to ward off the ice pick aimed at his head.

We were in pitch-black darkness in the middle of Lake Powell with no medical help available for miles, but fortunately John was not hurt. It took considerable time for me to calm Joyce and make her realize that murder was not the solution! She had been aware of John's many infidelities with some of his insurance lovelies and his latest dalliance with Julie was the last straw.

This incident put a bit of a damper on the things, but after several Bloody Marys the gang went back to sunbathing, swimming, and much more drinking!

Not long after the Lake Powell debacle, John and Joyce divorced. John gained custody of their African gray parrot, Tolbot.

Several years after John's divorce, we did another houseboat week. Much the same group went, but this time no Julie! John brought Ingrid, his latest significant other, one of his lovely insurance ladies.

Things went smoothly this time until one afternoon when we were swimming. Rosemary had said, "The nudes to the left, and the prudes to the right." Fast Eddie, one of the prudes, said he wanted to see Rosemary in her birthday suit. Eddie's wife, Judy, was not happy about that and chased him off his vantage point wielding a butcher knife! Fast Eddie barely escaped emasculation!

After this final episode, Rosemary and I decided that house boating, living in a confined area with too much booze, was not for us.

Nonetheless—on another occasion when Rosemary had gone to visit her aging father in Montréal—John, Ingrid, Julie and I visited Lake Powell again. Lake Powell can be a very treacherous lake with rapidly changing weather. Drownings happen every year, almost without exception.

John brought his bass boat and we took off for Rainbow Bridge, a marina several hours away. We arrived there for lunch and the weather was perfect, but just after lunch the wind suddenly became strong and the lake very choppy. One of the cruise boats carrying a group of sight-

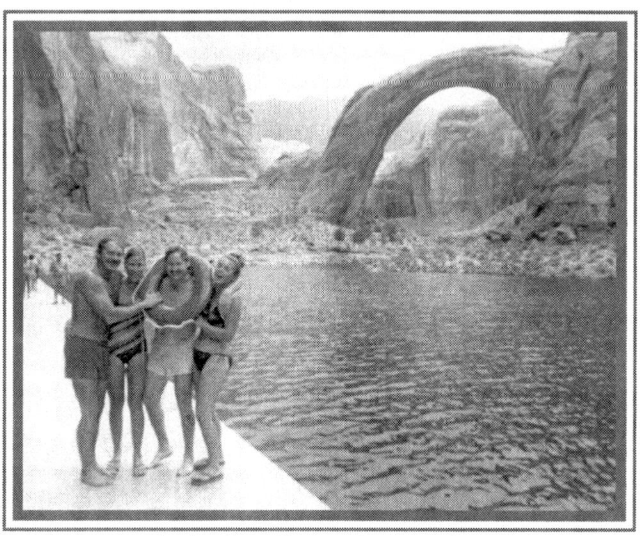

Lake Powell, Rainbow Bridge

seeing passengers was just leaving Rainbow Bridge Marina, so we decided to follow it in its smooth wake.

A bass boat has very low clearance from the water and somehow the wake from this large tourist boat suddenly swamped us. Although we bailed water like hell, our small boat was filling fast. We did not have life jackets. As luck would have it, we came upon a small ranger station at Dangling Rope, and we were rescued.

We spent a very wet, cold night in the ranger station. The next day the weather was considerably improved and we returned to Wahweep marina.

We stopped briefly at John's home. Talbot, the African gray parrot, had got out of his cage and made a meal of the telephone wire connections! In addition, the whole house looked like the bottom of Talbot's cage!

That was twenty-five years ago. Talbot is still very much alive and living happily with John and his wife, Ingrid.

Rosemary and I decided to buy a house, even though living in a high rise had been pleasant. It was Memorial Day weekend in 1980, and we were having lunch at a friend's home in Paradise Valley, Arizona.

The home of our friend was nestled with a small group of other homes at the foot of Camelback Mountain in an oasis-like setting just adjacent to the old landmark, five-star Marriott Mountain Shadows Hotel. Homeowners had use of the nearby hotel's swimming pools, Jacuzzis, tennis courts, and an executive golf course. The common grounds of the community were home to rabbits, quails, and roadrunners—and the occasional rattlesnake and coyote.

It was the silent serenity and beauty of the place, and the convenient distance to both Scottsdale and Phoenix, that impressed Rosemary and me—very much a feeling of being in the country, yet near the city.

Before lunch at our friends' house, I had several scotches and polished off at least half a bottle of delicious red wine. While many of my unwise decisions were made under the influence of alcohol, some of my wisest ones were as well. Such was the case that day.

There was a house for sale on the common ground. We met with the owners, Peter and Matilda Brand, and decided to purchase their house! It has proven to be one of my wiser decisions.

The Brands were in their late eighties. They had once lived in Hollywood, California in the early days of movies, and were friends of the late Wallace Beery who often played the bad man in movie roles.

Rosemary and I were invited to the Brand's home for their sixtieth wedding anniversary party, held in the home we subsequently purchased. Wallace Berry's wife (who was the very first Miss America!) had Alzheimer's, and was brought to the party in a dressing gown from the nursing home where she lived. Mrs. Berry was still a very good looking woman despite her age, but one would have thought the nursing home might have at least put her in a pretty dress for the party!

Peter Brand was a real character and an extremely lecherous old devil. He visited my office one lunch hour. Mary, my nurse, thought Peter might be a new patient, but she soon learned otherwise. Peter invited Mary to fly to Paris with him—she politely listened as he gave her this proposal:

"Mary, you and I will fly first class on Air France to Paris next week. We will only be away two weeks, and in Paris we will stay in the penthouse suite at the George V Hotel.

You, sweet Mary, will have a limitless shopping account and purchase anything your little heart desires at any of the finest shops in Paris. Money is no problem.

In the evening, we will dine at Maxines. Champagne and caviar will be the start of one of Maxines' famous five-star meals—a meal, dear child, you will always remember!

Later that evening, we will return to our hotel suite to retire. You will put on a gorgeous see-through negligee which I will buy for you. Now, do you know what will happen next? I will tell you. (15 seconds of pause.) Nothing!"

There was a rumor that Peter, in his younger days, had been a porno movie king. He was certainly one of the more memorable characters I ever met!

I was now teaching family practice residents (students) while carrying on my own practice. The residents followed me around my office to get first-hand observance of how I did things.

This may sound mundane, but I always advise my residents that after they have greeted their patient it is courteous to apologize if the patient had been kept waiting. Often the doctor does keep the patient waiting, sometimes for a very long time, and seldom if ever apologizes (Napoleon complex?)

This inconsiderate practice by doctors to keep a patient waiting aggravates the hell out of me, and I am sure it does other patients as well. "I am so sorry to have kept you waiting" are magic words, usually having a calming effect on a disgruntled patient.

Dress professionally, and always wash your hands before examining the patient! Preferably, let the patients see you doing this while apologizing.

Do not walk around with a button on your lapel that says, "I care." Show them!"

The importance of a patient's history and the physical examination must be emphasized. One of the foremost reasons why doctors end up in litigation is their failure to diagnose significant pathology—a malig-

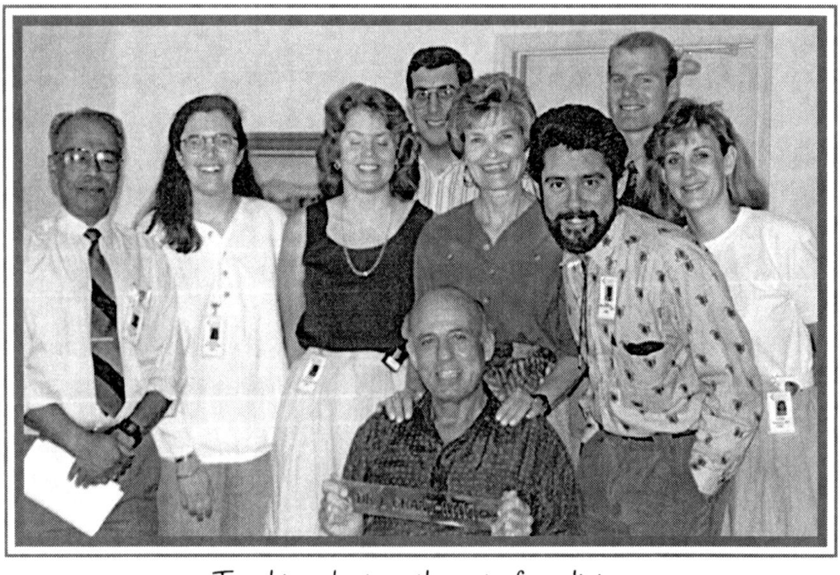

Teaching doctors the art of medicine

nancy, cardiac condition, or just about anything else. A failure to diagnose can result in harm or death.

On the subject of harming the patient, it is remarkable how many experienced doctors love to prescribe medications which have only recently received FDA approval. Even with FDA approval, many recent drugs have been withdrawn due to harmful side effects, including death.

I prefer to wait at least a year before prescribing a new medication. Invariably, other medications are available that have stood the test of time, and should be prescribed in the interim. Drug companies may not agree with me!

By carefully listening to a patient, the doctor is often able to have a good idea of the diagnosis or at the very least have a differential diagnosis (several possibilities).

Listening to a patient while performing an examination requires the doctor's undivided attention. No interruptions or telephone calls (except for a life-and-death emergency), no conversations with stockbrokers, no domestic calls. Such interruptions distract the doctor and can result in possibly missing something of great importance.

An example of such an interruption could be the doctor who is examining a woman's breasts, and is called to the telephone. The call may be from the Internal Revenue Service. The doctor may have just finished examining a patient's left breast, and returns to the patient most distracted. He examines the same left breast, believing it to be the breast he had not yet examined.

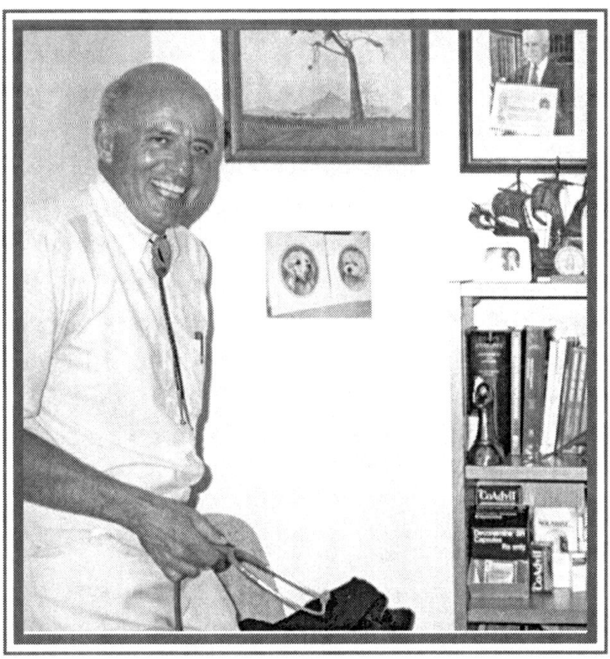

My consulting room

While this may seem an honest mistake, the unexamined breast could very well harbor a malignancy.

Patients should not be shy about speaking up if such a scene occurs while in the doctor's office. You are there for preventive medicine, not to have your doctor attend to his income tax or family problems!

The physical examination of a woman's breasts can produce erroneous results, especially if a lump is small, the breasts large, or mammography negative. If a woman comes to my office with a chest cold, not only will I listen to her chest but also I will re-examine her breasts even though I might have examined them a week previously. A chest cold is unlikely to kill you, but a lump that turns out to be a malignancy undiscovered on the previous examination possibly will!

By a thorough examination, I mean thorough. Many doctors have not been adequately trained, or are in too much of a hurry to do thorough physical examinations. How can you possibly find a melanoma in the left nostril if you do not look there? How can you possibly palpate a spleen if you do not probe deeply enough and have the patient positioned properly?

I have often heard patients (particularly new patients) say to me that they have never had such a thorough physical examination. This is certainly ego boosting, of far more importance is the fact that a conscientious history-taking and physical can often reveal pathology at an early stage.

Judicious testing, whether sophisticated lab tests, x-rays, MRI's, CT scans or other carefully thought-out diagnostic procedures may well be needed. However, over-reliance on the results of these procedures can be most detrimental to the patient and get doctors into hot water.

An excellent example of this is mammography. A patient of mine came to me many years ago saying that she thought she could feel a lump in her breast. I meticulously examined both breasts and axillae (arm pits), looking for pathological glands. I could not feel anything suspicious, and the mammogram was negative. This was long before MRI's. I asked her to return in three months for a follow-up visit.

She did not return until four months later with a totally unrelated gynecology problem, with out an appointment. I squeezed her in between patients and did not examine her breasts, but referred her to a gynecologist.

That same morning, the gynecologist telephoned me to say he was far more concerned about the presence of a breast mass than her gynecological problem. A repeat mammogram was negative, but surgical biopsy revealed an infiltrating carcinoma of the breast with axillary metastasis (secondary cancer in her armpit). In the end, the story did have a happy outcome for the patient, and twenty-five years later I saw her on a golf course!

There is a moral to this vignette. I told my residents that if a woman comes into their office and says she thinks she feels something in her breast, chances are there is something even if it cannot be felt and the mammogram is negative.

It is so important for the doctor always to have a high index of suspicion. This requires meticulous follow-up (red flagging of the patient's chart). If she does not come in for a follow-up appointment, make sure that your secretary calls to remind her! One would think that patients should bear some responsibility for their own health, but human nature often dictates otherwise.

Doctors often appear mesmerized by the results of blood tests, x-rays, and mammograms. A good clinician, regardless of any reports, should consider this is cancer until proven otherwise. If more physicians adopted this philosophy, there would be far fewer litigious suits for failure to diagnose, and there would be many more happy women breast cancer survivors to tell a success story.

I was appalled when I recently read in an article on the internet regarding breast self-examinations. To quote: "It is acceptable for women to choose not to do a breast self exam, or to do it only on occasion." A breast self-exam can be, and often is, an absolute lifesaver. For heavens sake, get to know the "feel" of your own breasts. They won`t bite you!

The correct technique for self-examining breasts is vitally important, and one must be instructed how to do this properly. Standing in front of a mirror, notice any puckering of the skin, indentations, or new asymmetry. Then perform the same examination lying down.

Many lumps, large or small, can be missed by speedy breast examinations. Even thorough exams can miss lumps big or small. A conscientious breast self-exam may well save your life.

Subconsciously or consciously, a doctor might feel that if he does not get the breast examination over quickly, his female patient might get the impression he is "feeling her up." For both doctors and patients, do not let this deter you and do not rely on negative mammograms.

Potential malpractice suits can touch every day of a doctor's life. I always recommend to my residents that, without exception, their nurse should accompany them in all women's exams.

Family practice consists of many routine patient visits, and my children, Wilson and Julie, used to call me a "cough and cold doctor." The two cases I am about to recount are those which stand out in my memory over many years of practice.

Mary Richards was fifteen years old in 1970 when she came to see me as a patient while I was practicing on the Lakeshore in Montréal.

Twenty-five years later, after I had retired in Arizona, I received a letter from the Québec medical disciplinary board stating they had received a complaint against me from Mary Richards, now Mrs. Mary Richards-Gavadi, alleging sexual impropriety. The complaint stated the misconduct had continued until 1978 (when Rosemary and I moved to the United States).

The letter contained some graphic accusations, but never any mention of actual sexual intercourse taking place.

At first, I thought this must be some kind of sick joke, but it certainly was not. The doctor in charge of the Québec medical disciplinary board, a lady doctor, stated that she had personally interviewed Mrs. Mary Richards-Gavadi who had given a most convincing description of what had taken place over a period of some eight years. Since Mary had been fifteen, she was a minor at the time and there is no statute of limitation for sexual misconduct.

It was my word against that of Mrs. Richards-Gavadi, and it was obvious that the lady doctor believed Mary was telling the truth. This grave situation could easily put me behind bars and cost me enormous damages, if found guilty. Not a pretty scenario after thirty-five years of blemish-free practice!

My solution was to find Shirley, the nurse who had been with me at the time and who had always been at my side during any pelvic or breast examination. This was easier said than done, twenty-five years later.

Shirley had divorced and changed her name, but was still living in the same area. After all those years, I managed to ferret her out and, bless her, she came to my rescue big time. The cruel and groundless case came to a grinding halt.

But what if Shirley had left the country or passed on and had not been able to come to my defense? My memoirs might well have been written from the confines of an Arizona, or more likely a Québec, correctional institute!

I have not the slightest recollection of Mary, but in retrospect I am convinced that she was looking for money. Most people know that doctors have deep pockets, and most are well insured.

In speculating on what may have happened, mixed marriages often come into conflict when the individual backgrounds are so different. Sometimes demanding sexual relations at unwelcome times of day or in the middle of the night causes friction. These are possible explanations of what may have happened with Mary, a North American woman who was married to an Arab.

Mary may have had marital problems, and possibly had consulted a therapist. Delving into her "repressed distant memory," the therapist might have come up with the idea that someone had access to her genitalia such as an incestuous relative or a horny doctor. This scenario could easily account for Mary's marital and sexual problems.

While this is all speculation, the really sad thing for me was receiving a final letter from the Québec medical disciplinary commission or syndication, all in French, which I had to have translated by my French Canadian plastic surgeon friend, Alfonsie Cigarre. The letter stated that the case was now closed because "I was now retired and no longer a potential danger!" La Belle Province! C'est la vie!

On the other hand, the Canadian Medical Protective Association wrote a kind letter, stating how pleased they were that the case had a well-deserved outcome as I had been completely exonerated. The CMPA also said it was unfortunate that these false accusations had followed me not only out of the country, but into retirement. Doctors, beware!

Doctors of tomorrow and doctors of today, always, always have a nurse with you when examining female patients or you may find yourself in very hot water, or worse!

Every fall I gave flu shots to patients. One of my patients, Charles, a man in his late sixties, came to me for a flu shot. Cindy, my conscientious nurse, gave him the shot and at the same time gave one to Rosemary and me. (For the record, flu shots do not cause influenza. Do not have the shot if you are allergic to eggs, chicken or chicken feathers.)

Six weeks later, Charles developed a somewhat mysterious disease called Guillain-Barre Syndrome. One of my bright and talented female family practice residents had quickly made this correct diagnosis.

I had never seen a case of Guillain-Barre Syndrome. It is a disease with a paralytic effect on the muscles of the lower extremities. It gradually works its way up, paralyzing as it goes, occasionally with fatal results. I called a senior neurologist in consultation. At that time, there was a difference of opinion as to how best to treat this condition.

Charles was in hospital for a great length of time and his recovery was a very slow process. Meanwhile, I received a lawyer's letter requesting copies of his medical chart. I consulted MICA (Mutual Insurance Company of Arizona), my malpractice carrier.

There was an outbreak in 1976, or perhaps rather a cluster of cases, of Guillain-Barre Syndrome. One of the ingredients in the flu vaccine of that year was a swine flu component. It was felt that this could be a possible cause of Guillain-Barre Syndrome.

After having spoken to the Medical Director of Parke-Davis Pharmaceutical, the company making flu vaccine at that time, I was told that the swine flu component had long since been removed and that there was absolutely no evidence to incriminate the current flu shots at all!

My nurse, Cindy, had kept the number of the vial from which Charle's flu shot had been withdrawn, and it was the same vile that Cindy had used for Rosemary and my flu shots! Talk about the luck of the Irish!

If there had been the slightest suspicion of any harm arising, do you think Rosemary and I would have had flu shots from that same vial?

Under the circumstances, there was no case and Charles still wanted me as his family physician! Nevertheles, there was now a conflict of interest and I decided it would be better if we parted.

Since these two potential malpractice cases amounted to naught, my thirty-five years in practice has remained blemish-free.

There were several occasions when a plaintiff or defendant attorney called upon me to review malpractice cases. Some of these were settled out of court.

One case involved a well-known O/G doctor who had a thriving practice in Phoenix. While performing a hysterectomy, he somehow managed to tie off both ureters, tubes that convey urine from kidney to the bladder. When no urine was forthcoming after the surgery, it became obvious that something was very wrong.

IVP x-rays illustrated that both ureters had been ligated (tied off) as no dye was seen entering the bladder.

A urologist was called in to correct the situation and the well-known OB/GYN assisted at the surgery.

What happened next? The OB/GYN had the balls to send his patient a bill for assisting at the second surgery! A malpractice case followed, which could have easily been avoided if an apology had been forthcoming and no bill sent for the second surgery.

Unfortunately, the medical profession like many other professions has some bad apples, and greed is often the motivation. In this case, the "noble profession" should have been the "no bill profession."

Many cases came to me for review, but failure to diagnose breast cancer was one of the most commonly encountered.

Two such cases involved lumps in the axillae (armpits).

The first case was treated for boils and given phisohex, a disinfectant, to apply regularly until the boils disappeared. They did not disappear, and in court I witnessed the devastating results of gross malpractice. The unfortunate woman could not have been very far from death. She stood there skin and bones with her husband and three young children. If I found this tragic sight so sad, so did the jury.

An award of many millions of dollars was granted for expenses in raising her three young children, loss of consortium, and punitive damages.

If the doctors of today and tomorrow both, as part of their curriculum would spend some time witnessing what I have just recounted, I have no doubt this would greatly increase their index of suspicion. The slogan, "Assume this is carcinoma until proven otherwise," is one all doctors should keep in mind.

The final tragic case involves my daughter, Julie. (Details on page 113.)

There are so many wonderful organizations collecting money for breast cancer research. Until the cause of this cancer can be found and eradicated, a woman's only chance for survival is early detection. It is here that women and their doctors should be playing vital roles!

A patient, John Alcock, had advanced chronic obstructive disease (bronchitis and emphysema). He was a dear chap and I was fond of John. Over the years as I looked after him he had become progressively more short of breath. This horrible disease has an inexorable downward course regardless of treatment.

As I was examining John one day, I felt his hand caressing my bottom, so I gently said, "John, you know I am not into boys, so what is the problem?"

Gasping and wheezing, his reply was almost inaudible. "Doctor, I feel so horny."

"John, why don't you jerk off then?"

"Doctor, I get too short of breath when I try."

"John, you poor bugger, I have the solution for you!"

Having finished examining him, I helped John get dressed and we went into my consulting room. (There is a picture of a dinosaur on the door leading into my consulting room, placed there by my staff who felt that I was still practicing in the dark ages!) I always followed up my examination of the patient with a visit to my consulting room, to go over my findings and make any recommendations.

"John, I am prescribing a vibrator for you. Have no fears, old man, this does all the work!"

With that, I telephoned Walgreen's Pharmacy and spoke to the pharmacist. "Jack, old chap, any vibrators on sale?" He answered, "Half price, only this week."

"Jack, you're on. Please wrap it up in brown paper as I am sending John Alcock to pick it up shortly."

Many patients in nursing homes were unable to come to my office. The Juniper Green Nursing Home once phoned me to ask if I would take on another patient. As I already had several at Juniper Green, I said "yes."

It was a Friday, and after my office closed, I went to see my new patient. The man was in his mid-eighties, completely paralyzed down one side of his body, with a fixed staring gaze at the ceiling. He was fed by a rubber tube placed through the nose, leading down to the stomach, and had both his hands securely tied down to the arms of his chair.

There had been no verbal communication or any response with the old man for the last five years, a good example of the "living dead." I felt it was inhuman having his hands tied down and requested that the nurse untie him, which she did. She warned me that he undoubtedly would pull out his nasogastric tube, as he had done many times before.

How could anyone with such restriction even scratch his or her nose? I mean, damn it all, this was not the Hanoi Hilton! This was none other than torture!

The patient did, in fact, did pull out his nasogastric over the weekend. He also had an unexpected visitor, a brother who was a year or two younger. He told the nurse on duty, "If my brother dies of malnutrition, I will not only sue the doctor but the nursing home as well."

The nursing home phoned me, informing me of the younger brother's threats. I telephoned the brother, trying to reason with him but to no avail. "Under these circumstances," I told him, "I am unable to look after your brother, and I am giving you two weeks to get another doctor for him," which he did.

His brother remained alive for several more years, still tied down in his chair with nasogastric feeding—an absolutely tragic situation that I personally was not prepared to perpetuate.

Several of my patients were pilots, including Ruth, a little sweetheart, age seventy-five. In fact, Ruth had been Senator Barry Goldwater's pilot in years gone by, and wrote a book on Arizona pioneering aviation history.

Ruth was frail—barely weighing eighty-five pounds. Every few years I gave her an FAA (flight) physical examination to renew her pilot's license. Since she was no longer flying, I saw no reason not to give her a doctor's okay for the license.

But finally, after her last physical, and looking at her EKG which was almost a straight line, I said, "Young lady, I just cannot issue you a license this time." Without batting an eyelid, she said, "I had been expecting you to say that for several years!"

Ruth had been to the beauty salon one day, and had just parked her car in her driveway when she was mugged by a couple of young Mexican thugs. She was badly beaten, and I had to hospitalize her at the Phoenix Baptist Hospital. The bastards had pulled off her rings, breaking two fingers, and her face was unrecognizable.

The scoundrels were caught and jailed and were ordered to reimburse Ruth over several years. She died six months later, never having fully recovered from the mugging. Reynold, her husband, finally went into a nursing home. I would visit him periodically, and found him to be a crusty old fellow way into his nineties.

Diana was a patient who came to see me with a problem related to her left eye. She had been in San Francisco when the problem arose, and had consulted a leading eye specialist there. The specialist reassured her there was nothing wrong with either eye.

Looking carefully at her eyelids, I saw something attached to one of the eyelashes. With a pair of splinter forceps, I carefully removed a small object and placed it on a Kleenex where it immediately started to crawl away! This little crab (pediculosis pubis) had lost its way and attached itself to an eyelash! These critters normally inhabitant the pubic area.

Diana told me that she and her husband had been making love on a sofa in one of San Francisco's more prestigious hotels. So, you see, you do not always get what you pay for!

Roy was another patient who came to see me soon after we moved to Arizona. He was an only child and, unfortunately, had inherited polycystic kidneys from his late father. His father died from a cerebral aneurysm at the age of forty-two, which can be a complication of polycystic kidneys. Roy's brain scan revealed no such abnormality.

His father was an abusive parent with an alcohol problem, and Roy came to regard me as a surrogate father. The stepfather (who owned an aircraft company), did not like Roy and paid him $10,000 a month to stay away!

Roy was a talented young man, but because of his monthly income did very little with his life. He was a gourmet cook, and could act, often playing roles in minor theatrical productions. He was also an excellent photographer, and he often photographed young strippers he had met in strip clubs. While he never charged them, he would give them handsome portfolios of their nude photos conditional on his keeping duplicate copies.

Roy invited me to one of his photographic shoots at his luxury condominium. He had all the props, including red boas and ostrich feather fans. The models were all attractive, but many of them had serious drug and other problems.

Roy was a member of a sex club, and invited me to one of the Saturday night "dungeon parties." Curious to see what went on, I accepted his invitation. We sat in the Voyeurs' Gallery and looked down at a party in full swing. Men and women of all sizes and shapes, many not too glamorous, masochists, and sadists—doing mind-boggling things to each other!

One man I spoke to was interested in tying people up with different kinds of elaborate knots. All very serious stuff! This unusual lifestyle was certainly not my bag, so Roy and I left early and went to Morton's, his favorite steakhouse.

In time, Roy's chronic kidney problem and general health began to deteriorate. He was grossly overweight and a chain-smoker, to boot. I generally gave him the last appointment of my workday because he usually had many jokes to tell and would bring in some of his photographic masterpieces for my approval! Roy was under the impression that I gave him preferential treatment, but I treated all my patients the same.

His nephrologist had him on dialysis twice a week which Roy found quite a chore. Incredibly, one of his girlfriends from high school days offered to donate one of her kidneys to him free! The operation was a success and for the next year Roy did very well. However, his blood pressure remained impossible to keep under good control and his heavy smoking did not improve the chances of survival of his new kidney. The kidney was rejected, and Roy went back on dialysis.

During his last hospitalization, Roy slipped into a coma while still receiving daily dialysis. He died peacefully a short time thereafter at age fifty-four.

It is my firm belief that everyone should have a current Living Will. This document should be notarized and kept with hospital records, with copies in one's own possession and readily available. It simply states, "I do not wish to be kept alive if I should have an incurable injury, disease or illness, or if I should be in an irreversible coma or a persistent vegetative state."

Under the foregoing circumstances, the following procedures will not be performed: Cardiopulmonary resuscitation, mechanical breathing, nutrition and hydration, surgery including tracheotomy, pacemaker, kidney dialysis, chemotherapy, invasive diagnostic tests, transfusion of blood or blood products, radiation treatment, and shock therapy.

The patient must be made as pain-free and comfortable as possible. Many doctors are still loath to give adequate pain medication, even when the patient is terminal! I witnessed this situation when Rosemary's father, who was ninety-one, was hospitalized with a terminal illness. He was restless and in great pain, with no pain medication having been prescribed. I called the doctor in charge and asked him to give 100 mg of demerol i.m.

The doctor settled for 75 mg as he did not want Rosemary's father to become addicted! Harold died peacefully within under an hour of receiving the demerol. This type of thinking by doctors is nothing short of malpractice, and is all too common.

Equally important is a Durable Medical Power of Attorney in the state in which you live. The person given this highly important authority must be someone you trust implicitly and advocate for all matters relating to health care, including without limitation full power to give or refuse consent to all medical, surgical, or related health care matters.

This paper becomes effective in the event you are unable to make or communicate health care decisions for yourself. If you wish to avoid much misery for yourself and vast expense to your family if you should suddenly become incapacitated, please take my advice and attend to these very important matters without delay.

Professor Harry Whyte (1904?). In 1991, my father passed away. I never knew how old he was because if anyone asked him, he would say between forty and death!

Dad was a social animal and loved to laugh. He had a big heart.

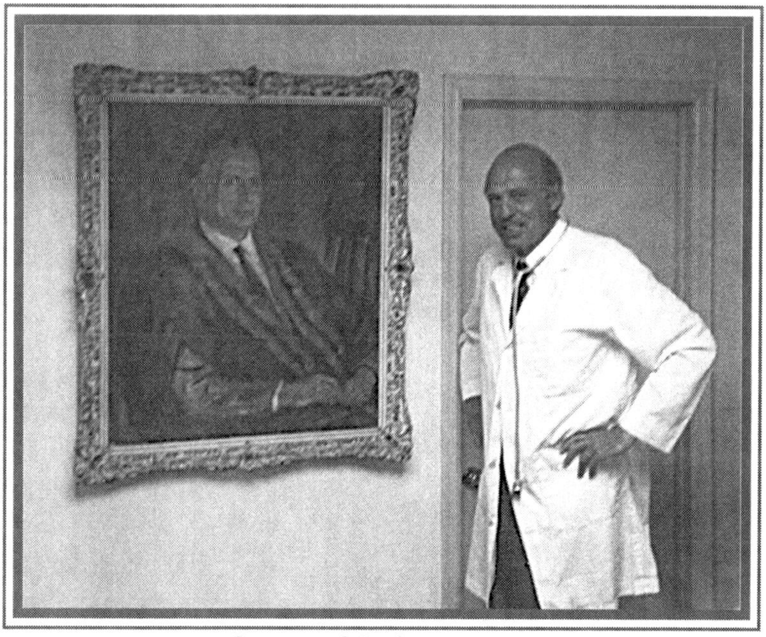

Portrait of Professor Harry

He was also a ladies' man. An incredibly hard worker, he was a highly accomplished doctor and received many awards of distinction. My father loved to travel, usually at pharmaceutical companies' expense as he was an internationally renowned anesthesiologist who had dealings with many of the top brass in drug companies.

It is safe to say that, when you consider his very humble beginnings, my father had come a long way!

Before I left for University, Dad gave me four pieces of advice. 1) Never let anyone operate on your nose; 2) do not get any young ladies pregnant; 3) do not get married before you qualify (in school); and 4) do not ride motorbikes.

I should have listened! While I was having my nose operated on—a sub-nasal mucus nasal resection (SMR)—in Montréal General Hospital, Lisa was getting herself pregnant with Mario's baby (possibly a thalidomide child). I had also successfully impregnated Lisa, and married her while still a student at St. Thomas'—a year before qualifying! But—I never did ride a motorbike!

You can well understand why dad was pissed off with me for several years. But it blew over, and we became the best of friends as the years went by. As you recall, he was best man at my wedding, and I was best man at his.

Dad visited us in Montreal, and later in Paradise Valley, Arizona with Norah, his lovely second wife.

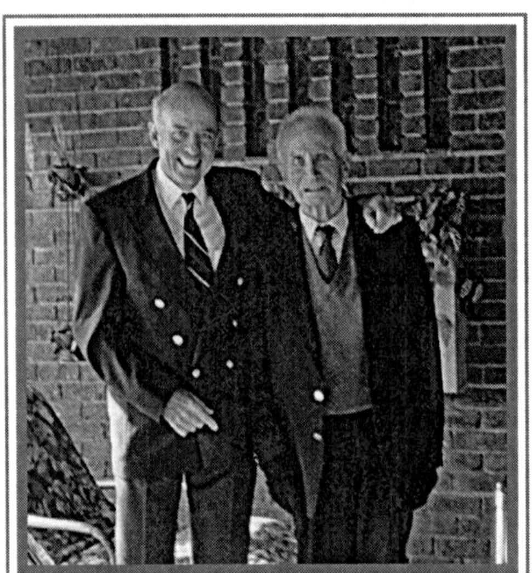

August, 1990

In later years, Norah became fed up with traveling and hearing his old stale jokes, so dad came alone to visit us. After a few days, Rosemary (who had also heard his old stale jokes many times) quickly took off for Montréal to visit her family. And so, during his visits, dad and I were often left to our own devices.

Dad often came to my

office and sat in the waiting room, chit-chatting with the patients. He had a constantly changing, captive audience and the patients seemed to love him!

On weekends, dad and I enjoyed going out to eat at favorite restaurants. When he got bored with my company, he would join other complete strangers at their tables. He introduced himself as Dr. Harry Whyte from South Africa, who lived in a tree! Then he regaled them (bored them?) with stories of his international travels and escapades (only the clean ones!). Often I had to pull him away, shaking my head and apologizing!

Dad loved music and while we were dining at Mancuso's Italian Restaurant one evening, he left our table to see who was playing the piano. The pianist was a lovely middle-aged lady named Margaret, who played beautifully. She and dad struck up a friendship and during dad's entire visit he and Margaret saw quite a bit of each other, literally! She seemed genuinely sad when dad returned to South Africa.

Dad wrote his autobiography, "Between Life and Death." It was a well-chosen title for an anesthesiologist who literally has patients between life and death. He never revealed the mischievous escapades in the book, but here now are just a few:

Dad and some of his South African doctor buddies flew to Denmark many years ago. It was a time when Denmark had live sex shows and this is something that intrigued the doctors because South Africa was well behind the rest of the world in many respects. When a plane landed in South Africa the captain would announce, "Ladies and gentlemen, please turn back your watches twenty-five years!"

The same group once went to Paris and visited the Follies to see Josephine Baker, who was then in her early twenties and a complete knockout. After the show, they visited one of the most prestigious brothels in Paris. This "venereal establishment" catered to voyeurs and other individuals who had some bizarre sexual aberrations.

Well, the doctors found great amusement watching through peepholes as some of their colleagues performed, and apparently little Tommy Thomas was a magnificent sexual athlete! Dad understandably omitted these saucy tales from his memoirs.

On one of his visits to see me in Arizona, dad and I joined John Temple and his harem for a weekend on Lake Saguaro. John kept a cabin cruiser at the lake to entertain his clients, his friends, and his employees. He was able to write it off this way!

It did not take long before we had some topless sunbathers on our hands! Josephine was a most attractive brunette in her mid-thirties, divorced, and had two children. I remember her well as she had the most beautiful symmetrical breasts, with a small red rose tattooed just above her left nipple. Dad was in his mid-seventies, yet he and Josephine hit it off immediately.

Dad was a "big fish in a little pond," but he had some friends who were big fish in big ponds. He attended the late President Gerald Ford's sixtieth birthday, and was lifelong friends with Senator Barry Goldwater. Senator Goldwater was one of the seven United States senators who did not vote for sanctions against South Africa because he knew sanctions did not work. My father met Senator Goldwater many years ago through his wife, Peggy, a most attractive and charming lady.

On one occasion, dad and I were the guests of the Goldwaters at the Paradise Valley Country Club. Barry was quite obviously tired, so after a lovely meal dad suggested I drive him home.

The senator had recently had two hips replaced and had difficulty getting out of my car, so I opened the passenger door, went round to the driver's side and, on the count of one-two-three, I pushed Arizona's beloved Senator Barry Goldwater out of the car by his rear-end. Not something many people can lay claim to!

Bertie Krantz and I once visited South Africa together where we stayed with Dad in Durban. I persuaded dad to come with us to Londolosi, a beautiful private game reserve on the borders of Kruger National Park. He came with us under duress, but was not a happy camper.

People come from all over the world to see the Big Five—Buffalo, Rhinoceros, Elephant, Leopard, and Lion (BRELL). We took off in a Land Rover with three or four foreign visitors just before sunset. It was a very bumpy ride and all dad did was complain bitterly in a very loud voice with every bump, "When the hell are we going home?"

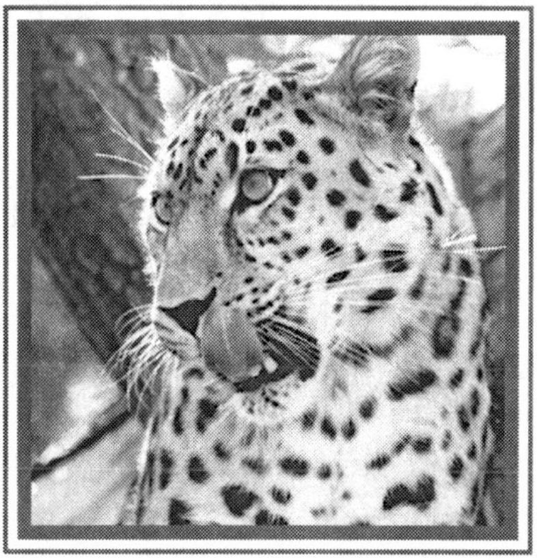

The three of us were having tea on a deck overlooking a large watering hole where the animals go at sunset to drink. Without warning, dad became disoriented and asked me where his automobile was and what had I done with his radio? He was having a TIA (transient ischemic attack), formerly called "little stroke."

I took him back to our room and did my best to calm him down as he was still quite disoriented. Leaving him for a moment, I went into another room when I heard the door slam shut. Dad had decided to walk home down the road in the darkness.

There were no fences around the camp, and just a week earlier a wounded antelope had gored a woman. I rushed after dad and literally dragged him back to our rondaval. I could almost see the headlines of the Natal Mercury newspaper: "Professor Harry Whyte trampled to death by drunken elephants!" Elephants eat marula berries and then drink water which allows the berries to ferment in their stomachs, causing them to get drunk! It was reported that during some of their drunken escapades elephants have sat on cars, much to the alarm of the occupants!

Dad safely returned home, and Bertie and I soon returned to the United States.

After dad's diagnosis of prostate cancer, I started to keep an even closer check on my own Prostate Specific Antigen (PSA) values (0.0 to 4.0). I had been keeping an eye on these figures for about two years. They had remained steady, but I noticed an insidious rise in the numbers: 2.1, 2.4, 2.8, 3.1, 3.6, and in the fall of 1991, the PSA went to 4.6. This is just a little above the upper limit of normal, but significant, especially with my family history. Father, his two younger brothers, and my own younger brother all had prostate cancer.

My urologist did the good old-fashioned rectal examination, and said he could feel nothing suspicious. He recommended an ultrasound and a biopsy just to be on the safe side, which he performed on a Friday. The ultrasound was negative, and the "random six" biopsies were taken and submitted. "Ian, they are all going to be negative," were the reassuring words I was given as I left the urologist's office.

The following Monday, Dr. Ian Nevins, head pathologist at St. Joseph's Hospital, telephoned me. His voice was somber and I immediately knew he was the bearer of bad tidings. He broke the news as gently as possible, but prostate cancer kills people and I became somewhat unglued.

Two other pathologists also looked at the biopsy slides, and they both agreed that it was an invasive carcinoma.

The Gleason Score runs 1 to 10, with the higher the number the worse the prognosis. Mine was six, the type of cancer one had to treat. I was now the patient, with a potentially lethal disease.

I can tell you firsthand that doctors are often difficult patients, and I was no exception. Peggy was a red headed Texan working in my office who listened for a few days to my ceaseless whining and whimpering. Finally, she bluntly told me to "chill out!" Advice I needed, badly!

The next decision was to opt for either radiation or surgery. I can fully understand how confusing the various options are that confront a patient with prostate cancer. After much consultation with therapists and surgeons, I elected to have a radical nerve sparing prostatectomy. By completely removing the prostate with its contained cancer, this would be a total cure. Radiation would possibly be the next step. (Not the other way around.)

Prostate cancer is a very silent disease and when first diagnosed it often has already spread beyond the prostate.

The secret then is to try to catch the disease early—often easier said than done!

The PSA can be normal or elevated in persons without prostate cancer, and vice versa. In other words, it is not nearly as specific as one would like, but it is a yardstick to go by. A positive family history and an escalating PSA could signify possible prostate cancer, as it did in my case.

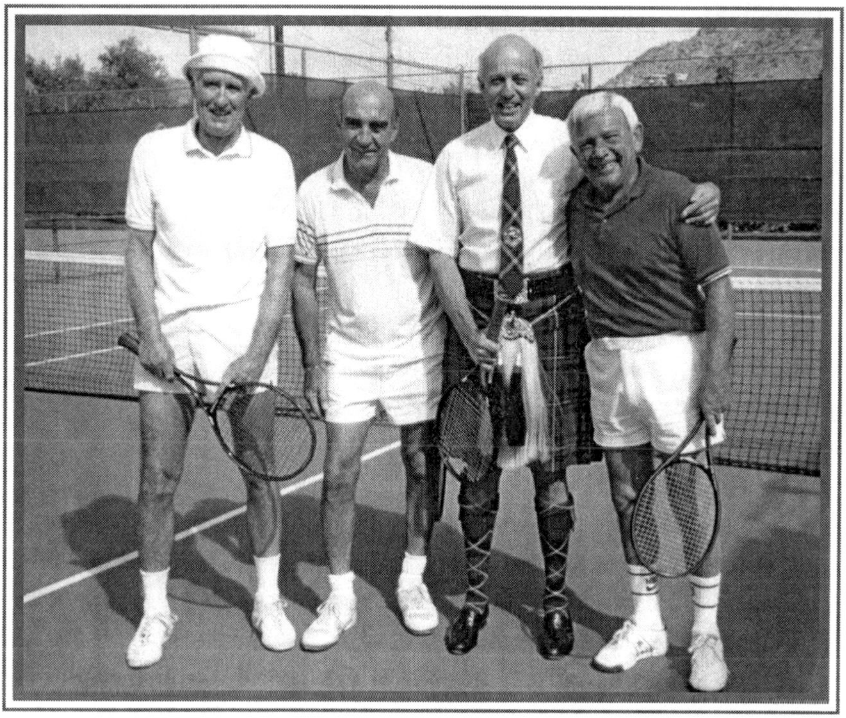

Tennis buddies

Biopsies are not without potential problems. To perform a "prostate self-examination" would require one to be a contortionist!

So, once again, your doctor must have a high index of suspicion with his male patients, especially forty years and older. Rectal examinations are still very worth performing and repeating. Induration (hardness) and asymmetry are possible predictors of a prostate cancer.

Prostate cancer is certainly a sneaky disease, and men should report promptly any changes in their urinary tract (blood in the urine, change in stream, and anything different). Again, it is always prudent to get a second opinion if you are worried.

One of my very noncompliant tennis buddy patients came to see me. Percy was in his early sixties, and during the course of a physical examination I detected certain hardness in his prostate. I arranged an ultrasound and biopsy.

At that time there were six specimens taken at random from the prostate (three from each side). The biopsies showed no evidence of cancer, but I was still concerned. I just did not like the feel of that gland. Three months later, I brought Percy back to my office protesting violently! "You doctors are all the same—just a mercenary bunch of bastards!"

"Mercenary Doctor Ian" repeated the rectal examination and liked even less what he felt. Repeat biopsy revealed an aggressive invasive prostate cancer. It was later removed successfully at surgery. "Percy, you miserable specimen, I have just saved your worthless life so that we can go on playing tennis!"

It is my understanding that today there are twelve biopsy specimens taken (six from each side), which increases the chances of finding an early prostate cancer.

A few days into recuperating from my surgery, I received news that dad had died. It took several days for the reality of his death to sink in and only then, when I was alone, did I cry.

Dad had an updated living will which specifically spelled out his end-of-life wishes. No machines, no tubes, and nothing to prolong life. He was adamant about it.

He had requested that his remains be cremated and that there be no religious service. These instructions were in the front of his regular will. However, some of his friends decided to host a farewell for him at the Durban Club in South Africa where dad had been a member for over fifty years.

My younger brother, Peter, flew out from England to attend the small gathering. Since I was still recuperating from my prostate surgery, I could not attend.

So dear Dad, wherever you are, I greet you with your favorite words of wisdom, the "Salutation to the Dawn."

I miss you, old man.

Look to this day,
for it is life, the very life of life.
In its brief course
lie all the verities and realities of your existence,

the bliss of growth, the glory of action,
the splendor of beauty.
For yesterday is but a dream,
and tomorrow yet a vision.
But today, well lived,
makes every yesterday a dream of happiness,
and every tomorrow a vision of hope.
Look well, therefore, to this day.

Such is the Salutation to the Dawn.
—Sanskrit 1200 B.C.

In 1993, Rosemary and I visited South Africa and drove to Pigeon Valley, a beautiful wildlife preserve just below our old home. We located the approximate area where dad and I had scattered mother's ashes in 1966. Dad had died peacefully from broncho-pneumonia, completely unrelated to his prostate cancer.

It was a windy, gray, and overcast day. The wind blew some of dad's ashes further afield, and I sadly said goodbye. Professor Harry Whyte died in the land he was born, and even the tragedy bird seemed to observe a few moments of silence to honor the passing of the big man in his little South African pond.

Oregon is the only state in the U.S. that permits physicians to assist in patient suicides. It is my understanding that very few physicians in that state had been called upon to render help to a terminal patient. Today, with the Hospice movement, active euthanasia would appear to be unnecessary.

Many doctors are fully capable of rendering excellent pain relief to terminally ill patients. To accurately diagnose when "the game is truly up" is not easy. In recent years, three of my friends have narrowly escaped the jaws of death, and had the plug been pulled I would not have been able to sit at their dinner table and enjoy a hearty meal with them.

"Do not resuscitate" is a heavy responsibility for the emergency room doctor, or anybody for that matter. With litigation rampant, doctors are often wary of not doing all in their power to sustain life.

Clearing out dad's things was sad. He was a man who valued human relationships rather than worldly things. I threw out Norah's love letters and dad's old photo albums—which I now very much regret doing! One of the old photos showed dad riding his motorcycle with a pretty girl on the back, in spite of his advice to me!

I also threw out dad's stockpile of self-deliverance material—succinyl choline, seconal, valium, and heaven alone knows what else. Mostly outdated stuff—enough medication to poison half of the American continent!

One thing belonging to dad that I cherish is an Omega Sea Master wristwatch I had given him in 1966 when my mother died. It is one of those watches you have to wind up daily, and each morning as I wind the watch I think of Dad.

Unemployment in South Africa today stands at about forty-five percent, and crime has escalated to an alarming degree. Rape, robbery, and murder are now commonplace. Johannesburg has become the murder capital of the world!

All of my remaining friends in South Africa have horror stories. My cousin, who lives in Cape Town, lost one of her closest friends who was raped and murdered after she drove into her apartment complex in Sea Point. Three African thugs attacked her in her garage as the automatic door was descending.

In another incident, Dr. Grant, a Pembroke Cambridge graduate and brilliant neurologist, had just been transferred from Cape Town to Johannesburg when he was murdered, leaving a wife and five children.

Another doctor was murdered and his car was stolen just north of Durban as he drove in to the parking lot of a hospital where he was to perform an emergency appendectomy.

Government corruption is rampant, as well, and there is poor or nonexistent administration in nearly all government departments. Many state and provincial hospitals are already showing signs of collapse.

Patients are not provided with food or bedding, and often no nursing care.

South African nurses are being increasingly lured overseas where opportunities are so much better. Education is also floundering. There has been a tremendous exodus of skilled people from South Africa, and an estimated half-million South Africans now live and work in London.

The races in South Africa are more polarized today than at any time in the past. It is now payback time for forty years of apartheid, and good reason to cry for the country, South Africa. It is a blessing that Alan Paton, who wrote the book, "Cry the Beloved Country," is not here to witness the disastrous path South Africa is taking. His book sold over fifteen million copies, and was translated into more than twenty languages. He worked all of his life for black majority rule.

Leaving South Africa, Rosemary and I visited Botswana.

The Okavango Delta, with wet and dry camps, was like the Serengeti of fifty years ago. In order to land a small aircraft, one had to buzz the runway to chase away herds of animals, the big five—buffalo, rhino, elephants, leopards, and lions.

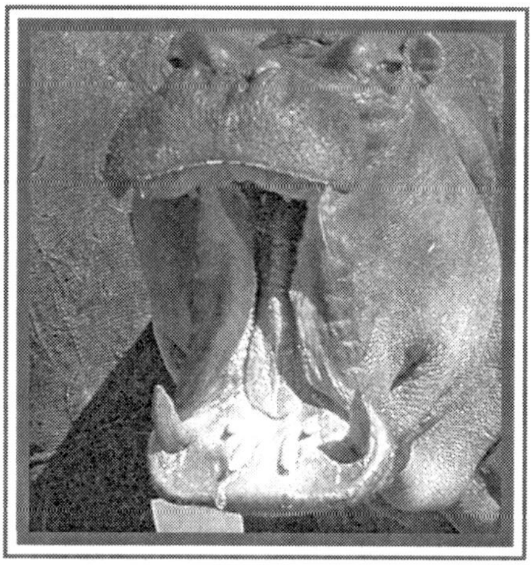

The hippopotamus kills more people in Africa than any other.

The Okavango Delta has been called Africa's last Eden! The area is totally unspoiled, with only few tourists. It was in the wet camp where Rosemary and I made a startling discovery one morning. Coming out of our rondaval accommodation, right in front of the front door was the unmistakable footprint of a colossal hippopotamus. The hippopotamus kills more people in Africa than any other animal. They come out of the water at night and stand on the side of the shore or on a road and since they are black, native people

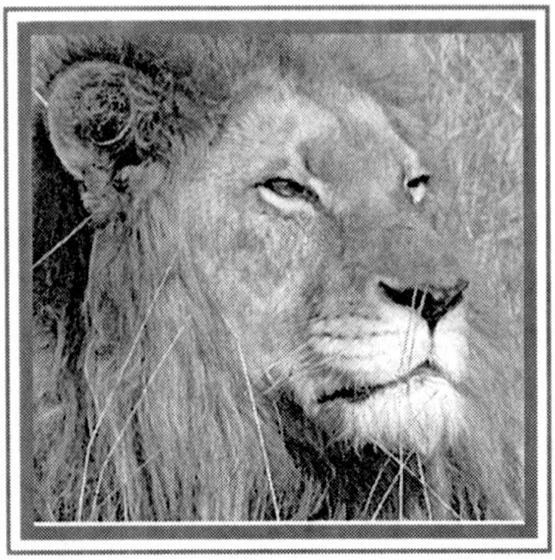

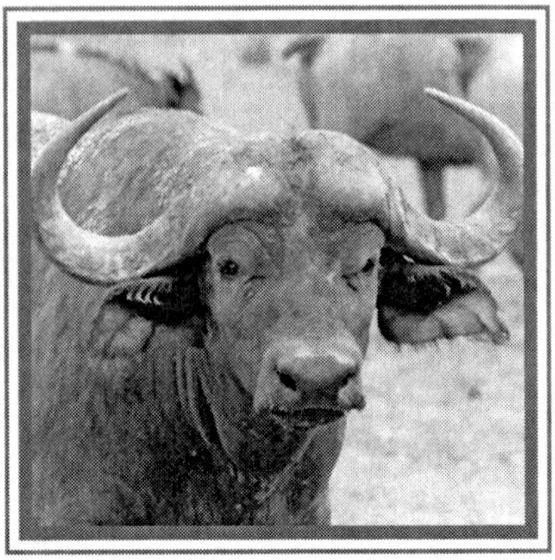

bump into them. The hippo instinctively turns around and bites the poor devils in half.

We saw a little boat with the entire back bitten off, including the outboard motor. In the Okavango Delta, animals have the right-of-way. You had better look where you are going!

A game warden showed Rosemary and me colored photo slides of a postmortem (autopsy) on a crocodile that had killed and eaten a black woman. Body parts and clothing were still discernable—all very frightening. The crocodile drags the victim under the bank, leaving him or her there for a few days before returning to finish off his meal.

On our return journey to the United States, Rosemary and I stopped in England to visit London and Cambridge. We drove to my old college, Pembroke. The Master, Meredith Clinton, invited us into his study for a sherry—Harvey's Bristol Milk, I believe. Meredith, the sherry, and the place had changed not one bit!

The Eagle Pub with its blackened signatures on the ceiling was still a reminder of World War Two and some of the poor blighters who never came back.

We continued on to Scotland to revisit some of the places I had been to as a student. The new owner of the late Mrs. Stapleton's magnificent estate, Conaglen, (Ardgour, Argyleshire) invited us for a brief visit. He had turned it into a hunting and fishing lodge. The magnificent old

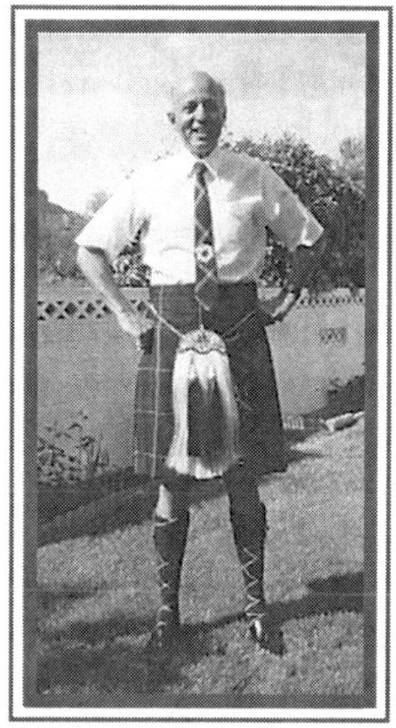

solid mahogany refectory table was still there where Mrs. Stapleton and I had dined, sitting at either end and finishing our scrumptious meal with huge strawberries and cream. The only thing missing was the pretty German housekeeper!

A stop in Ireland was next on the itinerary. Rosemary is seven-eights Irish, and we searched for some of her relatives in the cemeteries in Drogheda.

In our rented car we toured the whole of Southern Ireland, stopping one evening at a delightful place in Bantry Bay. It was a quaint Irish pub serving delicious food and some very strong beers on tap. From the sounds coming from the people at the bar, most were feeling no pain!

Returning to Dublin, the map indicated we would have to take a ferry, and so we followed the signs to the ferry landing. There, an enormous ship was docked with a long line of waiting cars. We waited for some time with the others to board, only to find out the ship was going to La Havre in France—a 22-hour journey across the English Channel!

Feeling just a little sheepish, we found the ferry we were looking for (which carried only six motorcars across a small river) just minutes away! Such is the confusion often facing tourists—all part of the fun, perhaps.

Back in the U.S., retirement came suddenly and prematurely for me at age sixty-two because of the diagnosis of cancer. A young Canadian doctor came down to inspect my fifteen-year practice, and bought it. Unfortunately, he was the wrong man for the geriatric-oriented practice, and many of my loyal aging patients drifted off to other doctors.

People sometimes ask me how I spend my time in retirement. A lascivious leer will invariably curtail further questioning!

For most of our married life, Rosemary and I have had dogs. Bonnie was a West Highland White that lived for almost seventeen years. Clyde was a Dandie Dinmont terrier. Our dogs were family, and to lose a pet was heart-wrenching. When the game was truly up we had our dogs euthanised, holding them close until their final tail-wag as they peacefully slipped away to doggie heaven. Each time we lost one, we swore there would never be another! (But there always was.)

Well, I can feel a wet nose nuzzling my leg, informing me that he needs to go out. Sir Clyde MacDougal of Glamis, (aka Mac) is our Dandie Dinmont terrier who turned nine on June 7, 2007.

When Mac was almost a year old, he was nearly killed by a Rottweiler. Rosemary, Mac, and I were spending a week in Ferry Beach, Maine. A Rottweiler by the name of HoBo lived next door to our rental cottage. Hobo was kept permanently outside on a chain attached to his collar and between two trees.

It was a little after ten p.m. when Rosemary and I took Mac for his nighttime outing. The sky was clear and the moon almost full. It reminded me of a beautiful poem called the "Highway Man." "The moon was a ghostly Galleon tossed upon cloudy seas, and the highway man..." No! No! Not the highway man at all, but Hobo, who had broken from his chain and had Mac by the throat!

It all happened in a flash. Instinct took over as I quickly grabbed Hobo by the collar. With judo-like action, I flipped the eighty-pound Hobo onto his back. I was kneeling, and my right hand was through Hobo's collar with my right arm fully extended. He was held in a steadfast grip, pinned down on his back with his four legs pointing upward. My face was barely twelve inches from the dog's mouth!

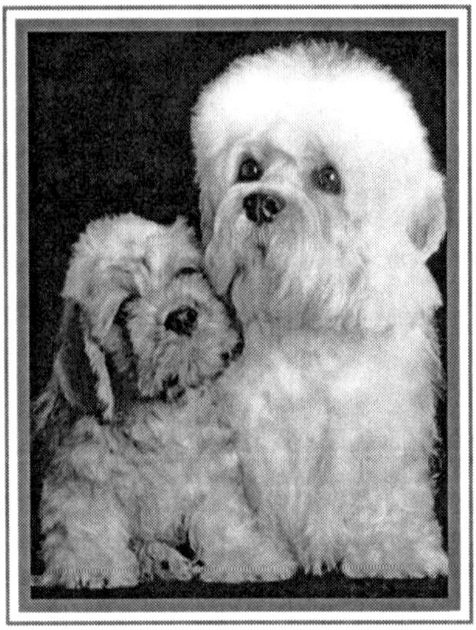

"Mac" and his grandfather

Meanwhile, Rosemary was yelling bloody murder. Hobo's very drunken owner apparently heard the commotion and finally staggered out of his cottage and pulled Hobo away from Mac. Fortunately, Hobo had narrowly missed Mac's windpipe (larynx).

Police and the Rabies Animal

Control were called, as this was an entirely unprovoked attack. Hobo had never been given rabies injections, and he was placed in quarantine for the next two weeks.

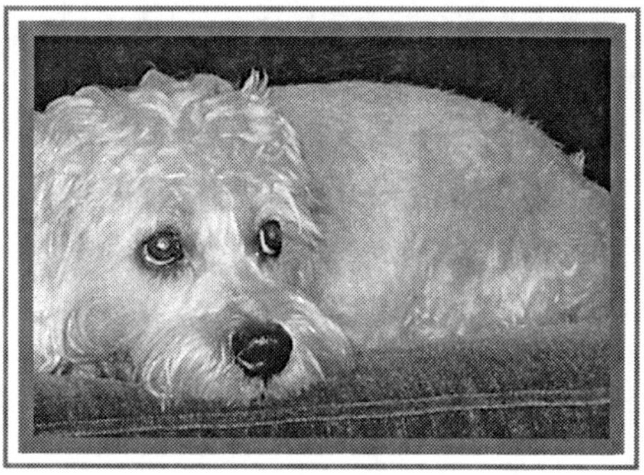

Mondern-day Dandies live to please themselves!

Hobo's owners soon abandoned their cottage and Hobo, leaving him without food or water for four days. In the end, Hobo was put to sleep by the local animal authorities.

People who do not protect and care for their animals should never, ever be allowed the privilege of having one! Hobo was not liable for his attack—the drunken, irresponsible owner was entirely to blame.

Modern-day Dandies are very different from the Dandie my late mother had in 1940. Most dogs live to please their masters, but Dandies live to please themselves! Mac and I were once thrown out of an obedience class for obnoxious behavior! That is, Mac's obnoxious behavior, not mine!

I have been accused of too often bringing sex into conversations! It may be true, because I do find sexual matters interesting.

The subject of sex has been exhaustively written about, so my observations are probably nothing new. However, I would like to address a few comments to men and women, married or unmarried, who are in significant relationships.

Caution is always prudent regarding sex. Nobody can possibly know what the (recently met in a single's bar) Wall Street executive with a fancy new Jag has in his "AIDS portfolio" hidden in his pants! Just as frightening, he may not know either in the early asymptomatic stages of AIDS.

In a bar's single scene, the combination of youthful immortality and a few stiff drinks will quickly see sanity vanish and hormones kick in.

One of my Cambridge colleagues was dating two woman physicians at the same time. One woman gave him gonorrhea, the other gave him chlamydia. Neither of these woman doctors realized they had the diseases (they were "silent carriers").

It is safer to have an ongoing affair with the Magic Wand vibrator until you are in a monogamous relationship. Just recently I went to an erotic boutique, "Roses and Passion," to buy a present for a friend. A young woman was looking at an array of vibrators. The one she ultimately chose was a formidable looking object with the appearance of an oversized black penis.

Vibrators come in small, medium, and large and in different colors. Prices range from twenty dollars and more, depending on the attachments. A very close friend, a nurse in her mid-seventies, always advises her newly divorced patients and friends to go out and buy themselves a vibrator.

There are many other outlets for sublimating pent-up sexual energy—sports, the arts, and a variety of interesting hobbies. In other words, a healthy, vibrant interest in life itself can diminish an overabundance of focus on sexual matters.

So get a life, if yours has become dull. Realize that life without sexual intercourse is not a death sentence! (I am not sure that I, or many other men, truly believe this!)

Not all people have the same intensity of sexual interest, and there are those who actually have little or none at all. Nothing is wrong or right this way. I once had a delightful married couple as patients. While performing a pelvic examination as a part of a routine physical examination, I noticed the wife was a virgin (she had a completely intact hymen). Questioning her about this, she said that neither she nor her husband liked sex. They seemed to be a well-adjusted couple, so there you see the other side of the coin.

Somebody once said that in a happy marriage or liaison, sex is but a small detail. In an unhappy one, sex or lack of it can also be a monumental problem. As couples age, their individual sexual needs and desires often change. The young sexual athlete of yesterday is now riddled with osteoarthritis. Sexual relations may have become painful, his good looks are gone, he is overweight, and gas is an unwelcome visitor!

The aging woman may have lost interest in sex. She is not the femme fatale of years gone by. Estrogen deprivation may be a factor, as well as concomitant atrophic vaginitis, dyspareunia (painful sex), and loss of libido. General disinterest in a partner of many years whose sexual performance, or lack of it, has become boring and monotonous, can all play a part. Sad but true!

So, what is the answer? Let me offer but a few. There are many ways of dealing with this common situation, of course. No one answer applies, but human understanding—compromise, compromise, and more compromise—is most important.

Unfortunately, it is often too late for compromise when so many unkind things have been said over the years, often under the influence of alcohol, and the relationship has reached a point of no return. Children leave, common interests wane, financial headaches, inability to separate for one reason or another—all can leave many couples in very depressing circumstances.

This sorry state of affairs should never have been allowed to get to such a point. Most divorces leave the combatants emotionally scarred and the children's lives in shambles. (Children are nonetheless better off with one good parent than two parents in a dysfunctional home.) Unless individuals are prepared to make fundamental changes in their behavior, life probably will be no better in a second marriage.

It is not surprising that so many people divorce. Different ethnic backgrounds, religions that believe sex is only for procreation, lack of communication, intolerance, and unrealistic expectations are just some of the factors. With common sense, caring friendship and companionship, couples can enjoy a happy and successful marriage. But it obviously takes a great deal of hard work, humanism, compromise, and most important of all, mutual respect.

Arguments often occur over the most stupid and inconsequential matters. One of my old Michaelhouse school teachers once gave me these parting words of wisdom: "Ian, nothing in this world really worthwhile comes easily." And that certainly applies to marriage!

These pearls of wisdom can never be repeated too many times. Never argue if you have been drinking. Do not go to bed angry, and always make up before turning off the lights. Never, never say I want a divorce unless you are deadly serious.

You started out as friends, didn't you? Look at those old smiling wedding photographs. Grow up. Say you are sorry! Let the words "I love you" work their magic.

When married couples both work, fatigue and stress can play havoc with sex lives. Make an appointment to see each other periodically. Put a smiley face on the calendar. Take the phone off the hook, muzzle the cellular, send the kids off to a movie, and most importantly, hide the remote. Spend this precious time communicating. Fantasizing is not a crime! Tell each other what you like, and what you do not like. Don't be shy.

A recent extensive survey on masturbation in males, between the ages of ten and a hundred, produced the following interesting statistics. Only two percent of males surveyed, claimed to masturbate regularly, the other ninety-eight percent were not telling the truth. Solution, just do it and keep the peace!

One of the lyrics from the musical, Hair, ("Masturbation can be fun"), brings back memories of my twelve year-old daughter, Julie, coming down to the breakfast table and singing this melodic tune. Mutual masturbation can also be fun!

The psychological sexual harm done to countless little girls in the name of religion is extensive. I believe this is something that has received little or no attention. The belief enforced in some churches that sex is for procreation only and birth control (other than the rhythm method) should be forbidden leaves no wonder that this type of criminal indoctrination may have left countless women with a lifetime of sexual hang-up's.

A magnificent example of aversion therapy.

Before leaving the subject of sexuality, I would like to mention a drug called climacteron. This injectable drug was on the Canadian market for over forty years, and was only removed on October 22, 2005. It was a mixture of testosterone and estrogen. The testosterone component had a profound aphrodisiac effect on many women and certainly helped ginger things up in the bedroom. Many patients were disappointed when it was removed from the market.

Perhaps one day a pharmaceutical company will produce a safe and effective aphrodisiac for women and men in need. Your dyslexic sex therapist has spoken!

On a Sunday morning in April of 2005 I was driving Rosemary's car near our home in Paradise Valley and drove right through a red light that had been on for 14.5 seconds. It was at an extremely busy intersection (Lincoln and Tatum) where many people have been killed.

This could have been a fatal accident as I broadsided a Lincoln Navigator at forty miles an hour. The occupants were an elderly couple, and fortunately, I hit just behind the driver's seat. Their car then struck a third vehicle with a woman and two little children.

Rosemary's 380 SL was twenty years old, and airbags were not available. My recollections are a bit hazy, but I remember steam coming from the radiator and my sunglasses smashed on my head when I hit the windscreen. Within seconds, a kind woman came to my assistance, yelling at me to get out as I think she felt the gas tank might explode.

The next thing I remember was lying on the ground while the Scottsdale paramedics and fire department were putting a neck brace on me. The driver of the Lincoln and I were then rushed to the hospital. The Lincoln driver had sustained only minor injuries and he was discharged the same morning, but I had sustained a severe concussion with fractures of multiple ribs and sternum (breastbone), and was kept overnight for observation.

The accident left me worried as I was convinced I had gone through the intersection when the light was still green.

I was not speeding and in no hurry, and it occurred to me that I may have had a small stroke. But what a hell of a place to have one!

I just could not believe the facts in this case. Perhaps there had been glitch with the photo radar? Requesting my emergency hospital records, I looked carefully through them. On the very last page were the results of my drug screen—negative for alcohol, cocaine, marijuana, barbiturate, but positive for benzodiazepine! Ah ha!

The previous night I had taken a dalmane 15 mg (half strength), a benzodiazepine sleeping pill at 10 p.m.—not so much for sleep, but as a muscle relaxant for my lumbago. The accident occurred twelve hours later, but the half-life for this drug may remain in the system for 24 to 48 hours.

The benzodiazepine group of drugs have muscle relaxing properties and in certain susceptible people (usually older individuals) a profound cognitive impairment can happen even after very small doses.

I am so grateful no one was killed or seriously injured. Regarding the woman I have been unable to thank who came to my assistance and kindly helped me out of the totally wrecked car, I offer a very belated "thank you" to that Good Samaritan.

Ralph was a member of my old tennis group. He phoned me out of a clear blue sky shortly after my accident, and said he had a business proposition. If I was prepared to invest fifty thousand dollars, he assured me he could turn it into two million dollars within a few years!

My immediate response was that if it sounds too good to be true, it probably is. A previous tennis friend had walked off with my first wife, Lisa, and now another tennis friend was after my hard-earned cash!

Ralph was always immaculately dressed and a seemingly successful real estate broker. He drove the latest Jag. I had known him for the best part of ten years, but never had any financial dealings with him. Curious, I telephoned his wife Priscilla to find out what this was all about.

Priscilla said she knew nothing of her husband's financial dealings and suggested I have lunch with him. And so, Ralph, Rosemary and I met for lunch later that week.

Ralph outlined how he and a group of investors had purchased prime real estate property very close to the next Olympic site. Somehow, they had received inside information on where the future Olympic village would be built.

Doctors often make extremely lousy businessmen, but this looked like an offer nobody could refuse! Doctors are not immune to greed! Should I give him the money now? "No, it should be sent to a lawyer in Flagstaff, Arizona," he told me.

What Ralph did not know is that I had him thoroughly investigated before our luncheon. This incredibly smooth operator had been in jail several times for real estate fraud.

He had defrauded a group of individuals of $29 million, and after unsuccessfully attempting to bribe a bank manager he went to jail for yet another stint.

Shortly after our luncheon, I received a call from the FBI and IRS. They wanted me to help them snare Ralph, who was not living up to his parole agreement and still engaging in fraudulent real estate transactions. He was also in deep shit with the IRS.

The FBI left me with a state-of-the-art tape recorder, a completely silent recording device. It was their hope I could get Ralph to incriminate himself, and the scenario was to have gone something like this:

While shopping in a haute cuisine supermarket, a young woman with a decidedly Southern accent would come up to me and say, "Oh! Dr. Whyte, I am sure you don't remember me as I was just a little girl when you last saw me, but you were our family doctor. Last year my parents were killed in an automobile accident. You might have read about this. Their estate is worth several million dollars. My parents trusted you so much, and I wondered if you could help me find a reliable, honest financial advisor?"

It is not uncommon for patients to come to their family doctors requesting all kinds of advice (a great mistake, if I may say so!).

Having fully explained these tragic circumstances to Ralph, I was then to give him the Southern Belle's phone number (a direct line to the FBI Phoenix office).

This was all terribly exciting, but when I discovered Ralph had many Mafia connections in Las Vegas, I quickly returned the tape recorder. The idea of cement booties or busted kneecaps for Christmas was definitely an offer I could refuse, thank you very much!

This amusing little tale involves a close elderly friend of mine, Rupert, who lost his lovely wife several years ago. Rupert is a tall lean man with size 13 shoes. He fits my prototype of a highly sexed lad!

We had finished lunch at Vincent's Bistro in Phoenix and, as we were leaving, a most attractive woman walked in front of us to retrieve her Mercedes from the valet. After she had passed by, I asked Rupert if he ever lusted?

His surprising answer immediately came back, "yes, every day!" He then asked me if I had ever been to a strip club. He never had, but in my younger days I frequented these dens of iniquity and vice on more than one occasion!

The Penthouse on Black Canyon Freeway was where we went. The young women dancers were very attractive, and exceptionally attentive. These places are terribly noisy and the two of us could not hear each other, as we are both somewhat deaf!

Within minutes, Rupert was experiencing his first lap dance. I watched in semi-horror as a blond bombshell did some incredibly nasty things to my friend Rupert. Then a frightening thought crossed my mind. Rupert had recently had a triple bypass. What if? Would I be held accessory to murder? How could I possibly explain this to his adult children?

No nitroglycerin was taken by Rupert. Instead, he had a second lap dance. When he finally came back to our table, with a giant smile, he told me what had transpired. The second, nastier lap dancer, "Goldilocks", was sliding up and down on his scrawny leg and mistook his wallet for—can you guess? A classic case of mistaken identity—warranting an extra twenty-dollar tip.

My friend, Bertie Krantz, was an absolute charmer. Even knowing he probably screwed Lisa was ancient history, and all was forgiven (not necessarily forgotten)! On several occasions, I tried to ply the details of his sexual relations with Lisa out of him, but he always pled the Fifth!

Rosemary and I had many fun evenings with Bertie and his wife, Carla. Both were gourmet cooks and great company. However, I never left him alone with Rosemary for any length of time! On September 23, 1963 Detective Caduc had once asked me, "How long do you think it takes, Doc?"

Bertie had once arranged for his married mistress, Karen, to join him independently at our home in Paradise Valley. Rosemary and I both liked Karen, and they had stayed with us on several occasions.

Absolute wild party animals, they had been smoking grass one afternoon and we could hear peels of laughter coming from the guest suite. Bertie came out briefly and asked if he could borrow some toys, including a bright shiny pair of handcuffs. Being the obliging host, I gave these to him and then joined Rosemary at the pool. (I did not want her to know that Bertie had our toys!)

Bertie had not only hidden the handcuffs, but had locked them to the large black candle fixture in our dining room. Initially he refused to give me the key, but later relented. Frantically, I attempted to unlock the cuffs and in so doing broke the key in the lock. Now what?

Suddenly I had a brilliant idea! My next-door neighbor was a part-time deputy sheriff who had handcuffs and obviously a key. I raced over to borrow the key, telling him that I had an old music box I could not open, and felt his handcuff key might do the trick. But the key was the wrong size, and at that very moment, Rosemary walked in.

Rosemary's parents were scheduled to come from Montreal the next week for a visit, so what to do? She came up with a great idea—take the candle fixture outside and paint the handcuffs black! You will find them there to this very day.

But this is not the end of the story. Bertie kept a black metal box with the addresses and photographs of his various lovers including a photo of Karen, spread-eagle and completely naked in our hammock. Bertie's arm was around Karen's shoulder and his hand perilously close to her right breast.

Carla had never shown the slightest interest in Bertie's black metal box, but curiosity killed the cat and the game was up. She telephoned me and asked, "Ian, how could you as a friend allow this to happen?" Not an easy question to answer, but I took a stab at it. "Carla, we are all consenting adults and if it had been you with your boyfriend, I could hardly have told you to go away." This was not going to placate her, and a long friendship ended.

Carla passed away recently and I phoned Bertie to say how sorry Rosemary and I were to hear of his loss. We have had so many happy times together.

On August 22, 2007, Rosemary and I celebrated my 77th birthday with Bertie in his lovely home on a lake in New Jersey. We had been friends since 1952 when we first met at London House.

Life today is good. For seven beautiful winter months of the year, Rosemary and I live with our nine-year-old Dandie, Mac, in Paradise Valley, Arizona. We spend the balance of the year in Montreal where we have an apartment on the eighth floor of a high-rise on West Island.

In our Lakeshore apartment in Montreal, we have over a 180° spectacular panoramic view from our balcony. To the extreme left our view is of Mount Royal, St. Joseph's Oratory, the Olympic Stadium, and Dorval International Airport where we can see massive airliners from all over the world landing and taking off.

Looking straight ahead from our balcony we can see the mighty St. Lawrence Seaway with massive tankers traveling to and from the Great Lakes, and to the extreme right are the beautiful Adirondack range of mountains, Mount Marcy, some sixty miles away. Montreal is an incredible contrast from the Southwest desert of Arizona.

We are convinced we have the best of two worlds in Montreal, Canada and Phoenix, Arizona.

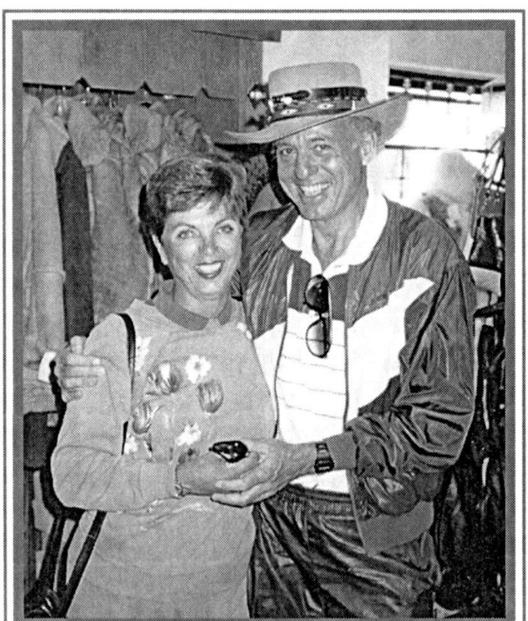

Ian & Rosemary

No More unrequited love; no more apologies!

Acknowledgments

My heartfelt thanks to Bryce Courtenay and Wilber Smith, brilliant authors, both born in South Africa, whose wonderful books have inspired me to try my own hand at writing.

A very special thank you to Jeanne JieAhn, my editor and up and coming author, whose assistance with this book has been very significant. Jeanne's beautiful memoir, "The Heydays, of Embassies, Foreign Adventures, and a Dog," was an inspiration, and I look forward to the debut of her next book.

Many thanks to Jim Aiken, whose remarkable photography and graphic design talents are immensely appreciated in the making of this book.

For Jamie Saloff, my deepest gratitude for her fine expertise and patience in transforming manuscript to book form.

Thank you, Juanita Copeland and Lynda Basye. Your individual inputs were very much appreciated.

Richard Guy, many thanks for your much appreciated computer help in Montreal.

Susanne Rothwell, many thanks for your map of South Africa.

Stan Rosenfeld, thanks for allowing me to print your information on penile injections for E.D. and P.E.

And "Dragon Natural Speaking" software, without their voice recognition program, these memoirs could not have been written!

To Contact the Author:

Visit him on the web at:
www.DyslexicDoc.com
or email him at:
grantwhyte@bigfoot.com

Addendum

Impotence

In 1998, Rosemary and I went to Italy on vacation, visiting the cities of Florence and Venice. Viagra had just come to the North American market, and I assumed it could be found in Venice as well.

I located a pharmacia just off San Marcos Square. Timidly approaching two attractive female pharmacists who were professionally dressed in white coats, I asked them in a very subdued voice if they had viagra. The immediate withering reply was, "Italian men do not need Viagra."

Outside the pharmacia, Rosemary stifled a giggle and said, "I could have told you that!" (Her previous significant other, Marcello, was an absolute demon in bed, so I was told!)

Since its release in March of 1998, Viagra became the drug of choice for treating impotence. In fact, I had helped Pfizer Pharmaceutical compile a documentary on Viagra. It certainly is a highly effective drug, but not without some potentially serious side effects.

Men of all ages can experience transient impotence, and reassurance is usually all that is necessary. However, it is more common in older men. This age group also may have co-existing coronary artery disease. For this reason, be careful before using levitra and cialis. These drugs can remain in the system for up to thirty-six hours, allowing older men more time to have heart attacks.

In a chaotic emergency room, the doctor may forget to ask whether a cardiac patient has recently taken one of these medications. The same danger applies to viagra, but it remains in the system a shorter length of time (about 24 hours). In any event, I suppose I am splitting hairs and there maybe many worse ways to meet your maker!

Impotence should be discussed with your doctor and the best remedy carefully tailored to your particular situation.

All information you could ever wish to know on this very important subject is in an excellent article entitled, "Managing Impotence—A Patient's Guide." This article is put out by the Department of Urology, Box 1695, UCSF Comprehensive Cancer Center, University of California, San Francisco, California. The article can also be printed from the internet.

Premature Ejaculation

Primary PE has dogged me most of my life. Secondary PE is also a problematic condition sometimes arising in men with previously satisfying sexual relationships. The onset of this type of PE is sometimes heralded by psychological problems needing attention. Reassurance based on clinical examination is often all that is necessary.

Premature ejaculation is far more common than you might suspect and involves ejaculating sooner than you or your partner would like. In my case, I feel it was one of the main contributing factors in my divorce. For ten years, I would ask Lisa if she had "gone to the moon" (had a climax) and her answer was always "Yes." She was a medical nurse, and yet could not openly tell me "No."

In primary PE, the most important factor in my opinion is the exquisite sensitivity of the glans penis (the fireman's helmet). One is born with a certain nerve supply to this area. A squeeze technique (stop-start), applying local anesthetic to the glans together with the use of a condom is a bit like making love with a boxing glove!

Masturbating an hour so before engaging in sexual intercourse may help. In days gone by, this was the sailors' trick before entering a bordello so that they could get their money's worth (and contact gonorrhea at the same time). None of these techniques helped me.

There are certain anti-depressant drugs whose possible side effects can delay sexual climax in many people. They are not approved by the FDA for the treatment of PE, but studies have shown them to be safe and effective for this condition and many doctors can be persuaded to prescribe them.

Find a doctor who will work with you to find the best drug to do the trick for you. (Many people are able to take these drugs with few or no side effects, but I must confess that I have never tried any of them myself because of possible dry mouth, drowsiness, or a decrease in libido.)

A combination of medications and psychosexual therapy will invariably help considerably if you suffer from secondary PE,usually a transient condition.

Be wary of a whole host of people out there on the internet known as charlatans, who make claims on curing PE but just want to take your money!

The "lateral coital position" was recommended by Masters and

Johnson for PE sufferers due to reduced pressure on the man. The woman begins on top (cowgirl position). This requires some "humorous" practice. If more people would only introduce some humor, fun, and communication into their sex lives, there might be fewer less suffering from PE and possibly far fewer divorces!

Let me make myself quite clear. You most definitely do not have to undergo prostate surgery to correct PE. The penile injections alone are often more than enough.

My first penile injection was administered by Dr. Barry Glans, my urologist. Lo and behold, my ambassador, who had remained moribund since my surgery, within minutes stood up and almost seemed to salute me! I was very pleasantly surprised!

I had a few errands to run that day and then stopped by Albertsons supermarket for groceries, still supporting an incredible erection. The young cashier must have thought I was behaving suspiciously as I had great difficulty getting my wallet out of my pocket!

This was the rebirth of my wretched old Ambassador! I finished my business at Albertsons, and like a child with a new toy I raced home to show Rosemary!

A short while later, I was scheduled for a hernia operation and realized that I might be out of commission for awhile in a very important area! I gave myself the magic injection but, for the first time ever, I used too much. By four o'clock in the morning, my ambassador was still going strong. What to do?

Since I had to be at the hospital by six a.m. for surgery, I was in a dilemma! Should I cancel the surgery? One can hardly go into surgery with a full-blown erection that will not go away! As luck would have it, multiple applications of ice ultimately did the trick! Try ice if you encounter a similar situation.

Penile injection may well be the answer for many men with PE. This type of therapy is essentially for those who suffer from erectile dysfunction (trouble achieving and maintaining erections), but as a byproduct it works magnificently for people with PE.

Jerry was once a patient of mine who boasted he could walk around afterwards with a towel draped over his penis! If you are interested in this, you can likely find a caring, understanding urologist to teach you this simple technique.

Hints, Questions and Answers

The following questions and answers were prepared to make the process as easy and painless as possible for men who decide to use injection therapy for erectile dysfunction or premature ejaculation.

Q1) After a nerve sparing prostatectomy, will injections help recovery of my natural erections?

A1) Yes. If your nerves were spared, the use of injections, which stimulate the flow of blood to the penis, may help the recovery of your natural erections.

Q2) What is the optimal time after surgery to begin injection therapy?

A2) As soon as the patient recovers from surgery and feels well enough to resume sexual relations, usually four to twelve weeks after surgery.

Q3) Will injections work on men with non-nerve sparing prostatectomy?

A3) Yes. Injections work independently of the nerves.

Q4) Are there different recommendations for injections for erectile dysfunction resulting from radiation therapy?

A4) There is no difference.

Q5) It seems that there are several different medications suitable for injection. What are they, and what are the trade-offs?

A5) Yes, there are several, and you should consult with your physician to discuss which is best for you. I use "Mayo Trimix," which has to be kept refrigerated.

Q6) How do these medications work to produce an erection?

A6) These drugs create an erection by relaxing the smooth muscles and widening the blood vessels in the penis. They are not dependent on nerve stimulation.

Q7) What are the long-term side effects with the use of these injections?

A7) One possible side effect is the development of a curvature in the erect penis, which can be painful and interfere with intercourse. It is called "Peyronie's Disease." You can minimize the risk of getting this condition by learning to inject properly, and this is not difficult.

Q8) Are there medical conditions that preclude the use of injections?

A8) Yes, severe scarring, allergy to any of the three medications, and active infection or sores on the penis. (Note: Blood thinners such as aspirin and coumadin can increase injection site bleeding. This can be minimized by firmly compressing the injection site for at least five minutes.)

Q9) What percentage of men will get a useful erection from an injection? Do injections work for everyone?

A9) If the medication is properly dosed (this is done by your physician) and injected correctly, a most useful erection should occur in at least eighty percent of men.

Q10) Does the medication continue to work indefinitely or is a tolerance created requiring increased dosage?

A10) Both conditions have occurred.

Q11) How long will the erections last?

A11) If the proper dosage is administered correctly, erections generally appear five to ten minutes after injection and generally last for about half an hour, or quite a bit longer on occasion.

Q12) Can injections be used with a vacuum erection device?

A12) Do not ever do this as serious bleeding may occur!

Q13) My medication requires refrigeration. How long can it be left unrefrigerated?

A13) Not more than three hours. Some medications do not need refrigeration, and this is useful when traveling. Consult your physician.

Q14) What is Priapism?

A14) This is an erection lasting more than four hours, and you should go immediately to an emergency room for treatment. Serious damage to the penis may otherwise occur.

Q15) I have heard that Sudafed and Benedryl can help reduce a prolonged erection. When should these be used?

A15) If the erection lasts more than two hours. A visit to the emergency room is mandatory if the erection lasts four hours.

Q16) Can I use an ice pack to reduce an erection? Where and how should it be applied?

A16) Yes, on the penis or inner part of the thighs. A cold shower may also work.

Concerning injection mechanics and the correct place to inject, it is essential to consult a urologist before attempting to self-administer a penile injection. The doctor can give you all the necessary details on where to inject, how much to use, and answers to any other questions you may have.

There is an auto injector available, which I have never used. This gadget inserts the needle into the penis very quickly, minimizing discomfort and psychological hesitancy. If you are chicken about giving yourself injections, this may be the way to go.

With injection therapy, you are able to last as long as you wish! I certainly don't recommend much over an hour. The beautiful thing about the injection therapy is that even after you have ejaculated your ambassador remains ramrod stiff, and it just keeps going and going and going! Amazing but true.

I can assure you that your efforts will be rewarded. Voila. Good luck.

Printed in the United States
104641LV00004B/274-312/P